Seeing Color Colorblind

Protanopia Part I

SUSAN BRANDT GRAHAM, MD, PhD

Formally trained in Anthropology (PhD) and Medicine (MD), Susan Brandt Graham is a photographic artist who has had a lifelong interest in understanding how "colorblind" people see the world. Using the art and technology of digital photography, she unlocks the fascinating world seen by people with severe red deficient vision.

Seeing Color Colorblind
Protanopia Part I
Text and All Images
Copyright © 2016 Susan Brandt Graham
All Rights Reserved.

ISBN: 153292805X
ISBN-13: 978-1532928055

DEDICATION

To BG and CHB

CONTENTS

ACKNOWLEDGMENTS	i
1 PREFACE	1
2 SEEING COLOR COLORBLIND	3
3 PINKS, ORANGES, AND REDS	5
4 YELLOWS	19
5 BLUES	27
6 MONOCHROME, AND BLACK AND WHITE	33
7 SKIN TONES	43
POSTSCRIPT	50
ABOUT THE AUTHOR	51

ACKNOWLEDGMENTS

Without the input, insights, suggestions and encouragement of Brandt Graham, my son, I could not have created the diptychs comparing images as seen by people with normal color vision versus images as perceived by an individual with severe red deficiency vision. The diptychs are the basis of this volume, a photo essay. We were pretty pleased with ourselves when we were able to accomplish this within the RGB color space of projected light on our computer monitors, working at a distance. Producing an informative and affordable paperback volume in the CMYK color space of reflected light required for print presented a special series of challenges for two very different pairs of eyes. Many printed proofs were required before we achieved what we had set out to do. We are proud of what we have done together. For me, the journey has been a high point in my life; Brandt taught me to see the world through his eyes.

Friends Tim and Laurie Price have shared not only photographic and artistic insights over the years, but have been companions on "photographic excursions" that produced some of the images in this volume. Lois Brandt, my mom, is a geneticist who introduced me to inheritance patterns at a young age. She has always encouraged me to write beyond the confines of peer-reviewed academic journals. More recently, Jim Stallings has introduced me to the joys of indie publishing. I thank each of them for their contributions to what has become a labor of love.

1 PREFACE

What does the world look like to "colorblind" people? What do they see? There is no single right answer, because different types and degrees of color vision deficiencies are found worldwide.

"Colorblindness" has always been present in my life. My father was "red-green colorblind." I never really knew exactly what that meant until recently. I just knew he had trouble differentiating some colors, and that on vacations he would ask my mother what color the traffic lights were. But he was good natured about it. When I was a small girl, I tried to "teach him his colors" using my mother's many colored spools of thread. He played along. I recall numerous times when people would ask him what color he saw in something, and he always gave an answer that sounded plausible to people who had no clue that it was all made up. It must have been easier than trying to explain to people that he couldn't describe a color he had never seen. I don't know if his color deficiency presented problems when he was growing up or not. He was a child of the Great Depression, and his father had died when he was three years old. I suspect his childhood was full of many more overwhelming problems than seeing the world of color differently from the majority of people, but none of those were ever discussed with me.

My mother is a geneticist. She knew, of course, that any son of mine would have a 50-50 chance of being colorblind like my father. I knew it from at least the time I was in high school. I do not remember exactly when we knew my son was colorblind like his maternal grandfather, but he was very young. In retrospect, none of us in the family thought much about it. It was what it was, certainly not unexpected. My father and son saw the world alike, and understood each other. They did not have to explain to each other what they saw. Perhaps the thing my mother remembers most about my son's childhood was his love of black balloons.

And, I'll never forget when my father was visiting, he and my son, only three or four years old, were watching a football game on our black and white television. I thought they were carrying out an elaborate joke when they kept talking about "the blue team and the yellow team." Since I did not believe they could possibly be seeing color on a black and white television, I marveled that my father had taught such a small child to be able to participate in the joke without "spilling the beans." The joke definitely was on me, but not in the way that I thought at the time.

Because colorblindness was such a normal part of family life, before beginning work on this project I had never considered the deep impact it might have had on my son, especially in the school years. If any parents with young children are reading this, let me say that there are good books out there about some of the problems children with color vision deficiencies encounter, and resources to help parents help their children deal with them. I certainly wish I had been more aware as a mother.

On March 15, 2015 I saw the first in a series of videos made by EnChroma, a company that makes glasses that help many people with color vision deficiencies see a broader range of colors. I must have watched the video at least twenty times that day, and cried throughout. I thought of the times my son had said, "I wish just once, even if just for a minute, I could see the world the way other people do." Finally, here was the chance, I thought. My mother saw the video, and immediately ordered some of the EnChroma glasses for her grandson.

Unfortunately, the glasses as developed to the time of this writing do not provide the "wow" effect for people with protanopia, or severe red deficiency. My son reports seeing a little pink with them, and he does enjoy the way things look overall with the glasses. He is very glad he has them. When I realized at that point that the technology does not yet exist for him to see the world as I see it, I began to wonder if there were any way I could see the world through his eyes. The answer was yes, through the use of photography and a variety of digital techniques I had learned over the years. My son has helped to verify results as we worked on these images. The process has increased my understanding of my adult son and his life, and, at least for me, has deepened our relationship. This is the most satisfying use of photography I have made to date - to see the world through the eyes of my son and father.

2 SEEING COLOR COLORBLIND

Seeing color is something that those of us with normal color vision take for granted. People with color deficiencies make clear that our senses, including seeing color, are individual. Seeing color requires photo pigments in the cones of the eye to sense long wavelength light (L cones, roughly "red"), medium wavelength light (M cones, roughly "green"), and short wavelength light (S cones, roughly "blue").

"Colorblind" has been applied to people with a wide range of color deficiencies in the required photo pigments. Deficiencies in red photo pigments and in green photo pigments have often been lumped together as "red-green colorblindness," but people with red deficiencies perceive the world differently from people with green deficiencies, and vice versa. Protanopia is a severe form of red deficiency. People with this form of color deficiency are sometimes called "red dichromats" because they have only two kinds of working cones, the M cones and the S cones.

Most genetic color deficiencies are inherited as X-linked recessive traits. The genes that make the photo pigments are located on the X chromosome. Females have two X chromosomes, while males have one X chromosome and one Y chromosome. Females inherit one X chromosome from their mother and one X chromosome from their father. Males inherit their X chromosome from their mother, and their Y chromosome from their father. If one X chromosome is deficient but the other is normal, the female usually has normal color vision. That is, it usually requires two abnormal X chromosomes for a woman to be "colorblind." The situation is different for males. The Y chromosome is shorter than the X chromosome and does not contain a counterpart to produce photo pigments. Thus, a male who inherits an abnormal X chromosome will be color deficient. This is why so many more males than females experience color deficient sight.

My son, Brandt, who has severe red deficiency like his maternal grandfather, has said:

"'Colorblind' as a term is sort of a misnomer in that even extremely colorblind people see colors - they just see them differently than people who are not 'colorblind.' Unfortunately, many people are ignorant regarding this. The most ignorant comments seem to generally involve references to black and white television…which is not in the right ballpark."

I set out to create diptychs in which both images appear the same to someone with severe red deficiency. My son has confirmed that these images appear the same to him. Skin tones shocked me, while things we see somewhat similarly pleased me.

The primary colors of light in the RGB additive system are Red, Green, and Blue. If a person is lacking the photo pigments to perceive red, then blue and green and various combinations thereof will be what is perceived.

These diptychs showing images as seen by someone with normal color vision and by someone with a severe red deficiency are from the first phase of a project to illustrate how people with different types and degrees of color deficiency or "colorblindness" see the world. Having lived my entire life around people with severe red deficiency and wondering how the world looked to them, this project became very important to me on a personal level. In some ways I believe it also became important to my son with a red deficiency. I hope it may in some small way help other families with color deficiencies. Many people with color deficiencies feel put on the spot if asked, "What color do you see," because in some ways it is a meaningless question. But, I do believe that many people would like for normal color sighted people to understand their world. Comparing images in diptychs is nonthreatening: a simple "yes" or "no" is all that is required.

EnChroma (www. Enchroma.com) makes glasses that help many "colorblind" people to see a wider range of colors, but they do not help my son. I hope that in his lifetime technology will be developed to allow him to see my world of color. The most important thing I learned in this project, however, is that the world of my son, while different, is beautiful in its own right.

3 PINKS, ORANGES, AND REDS

People with severe red deficiency vision often see other colors quite differently from people with normal color vision. White, which in the additive RGB system is the combination of all colors, may be perceived as cyan. Pink becomes a gray or a blue.

For the red dichromat, the orange reds become difficult to distinguish from greens. Orange becomes a kind of chartreuse. Even the green of leaves changes, because most have some degree of red in them. These reds in the leaves are not perceived by the dichromat, and this is why even the leaf colors appear different in these images.

True reds in nature are perceived as almost black.

Image 3-1   Desert Rose

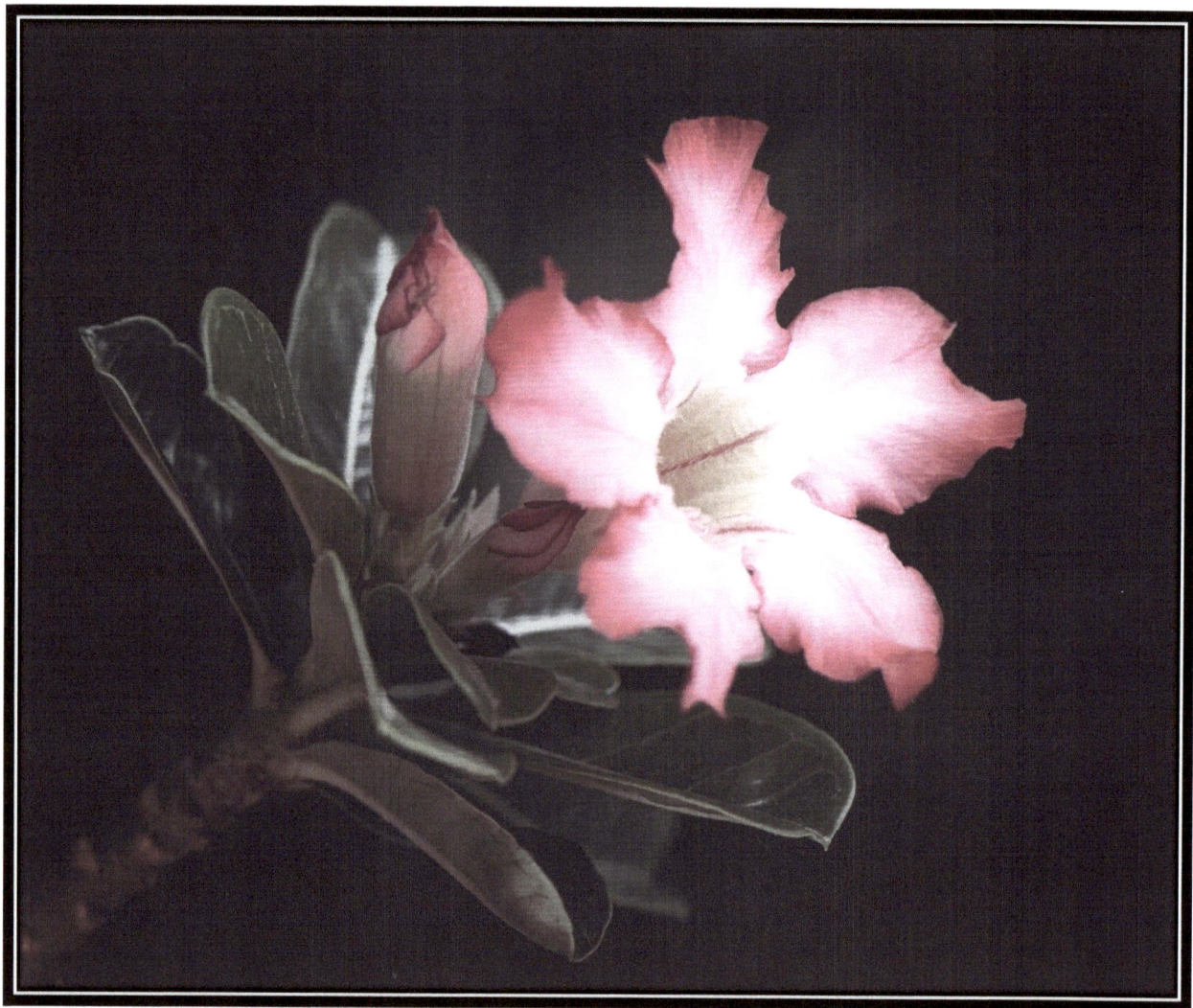

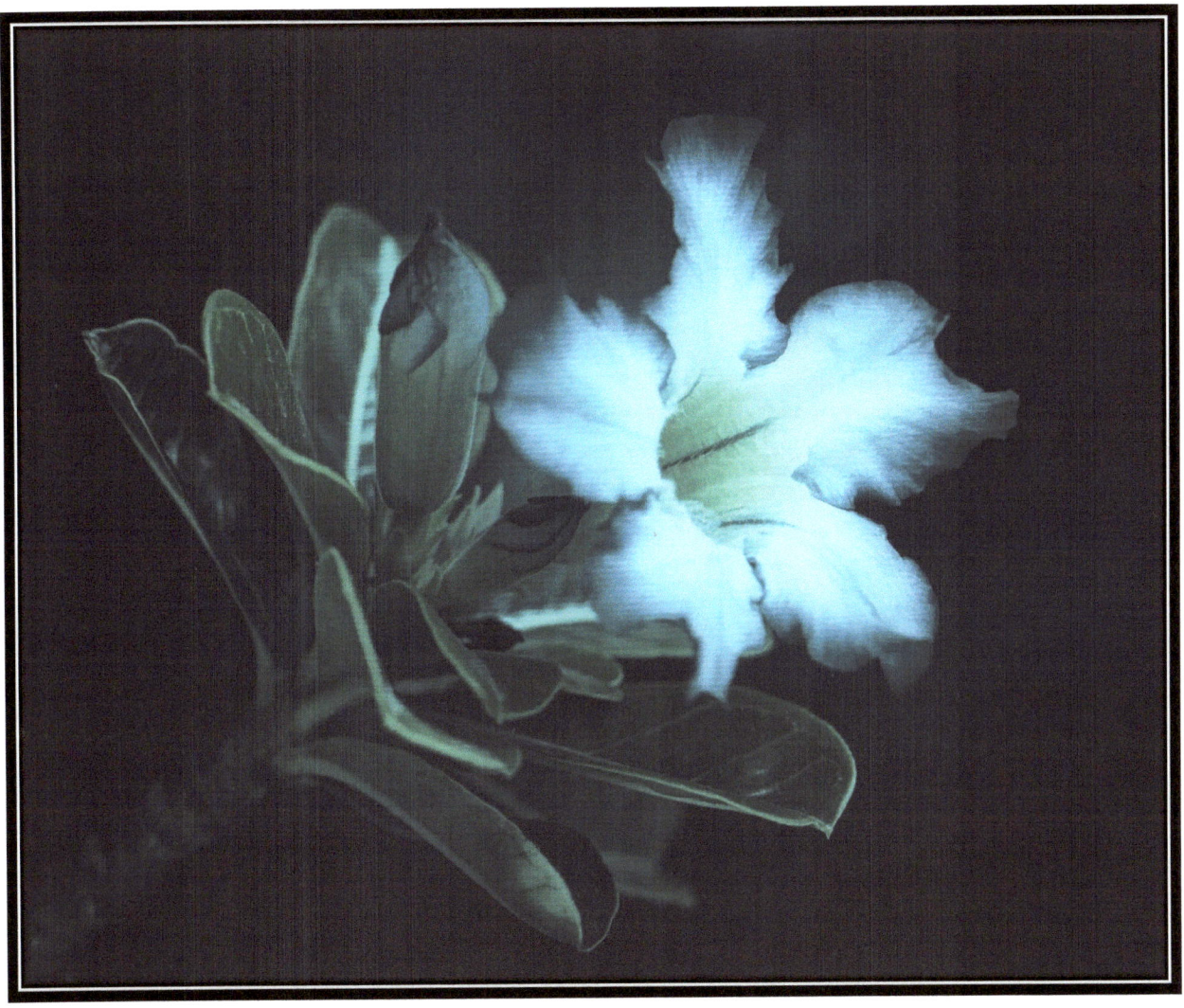

Image 3-2   Red Lacewing Butterfly

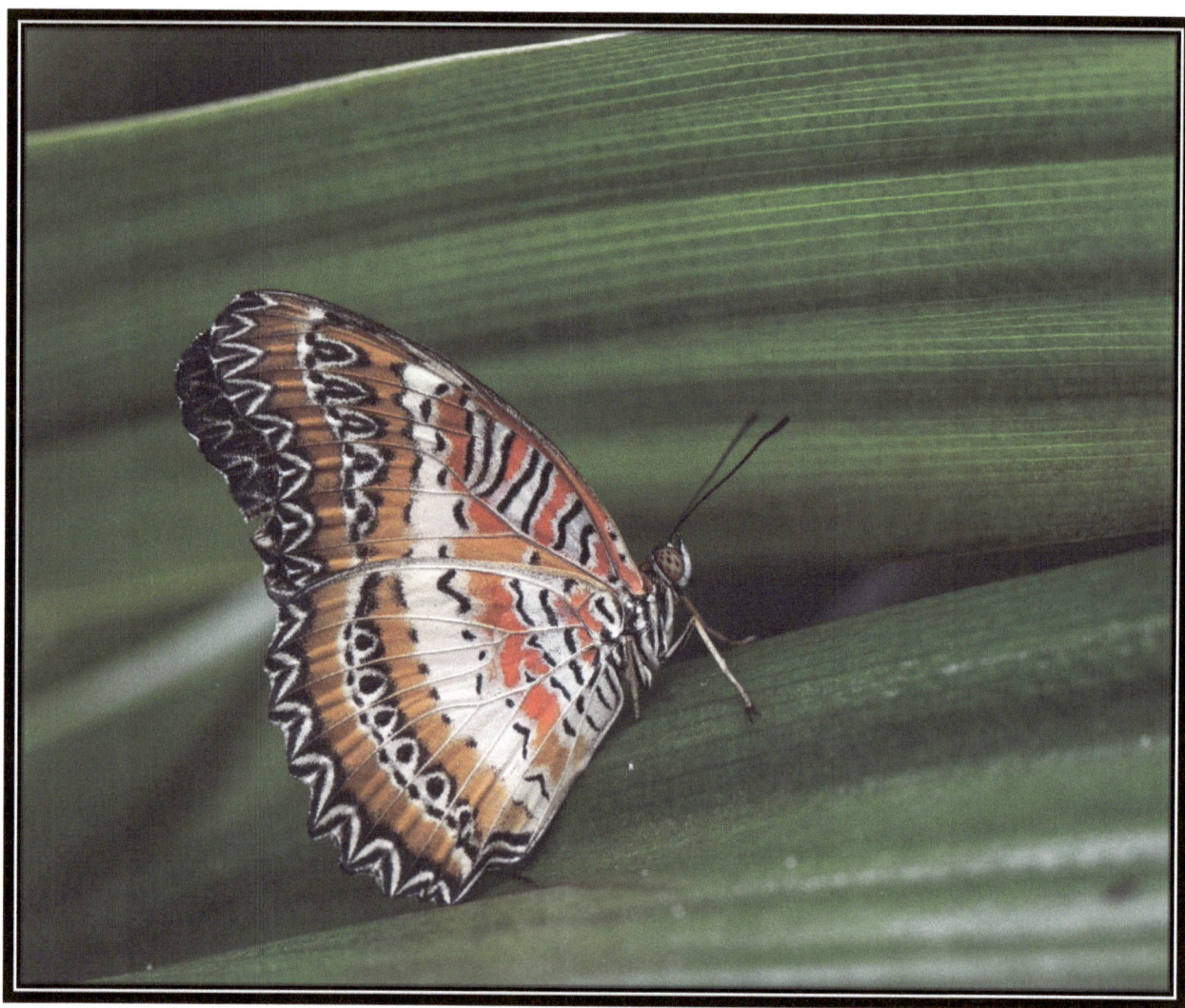

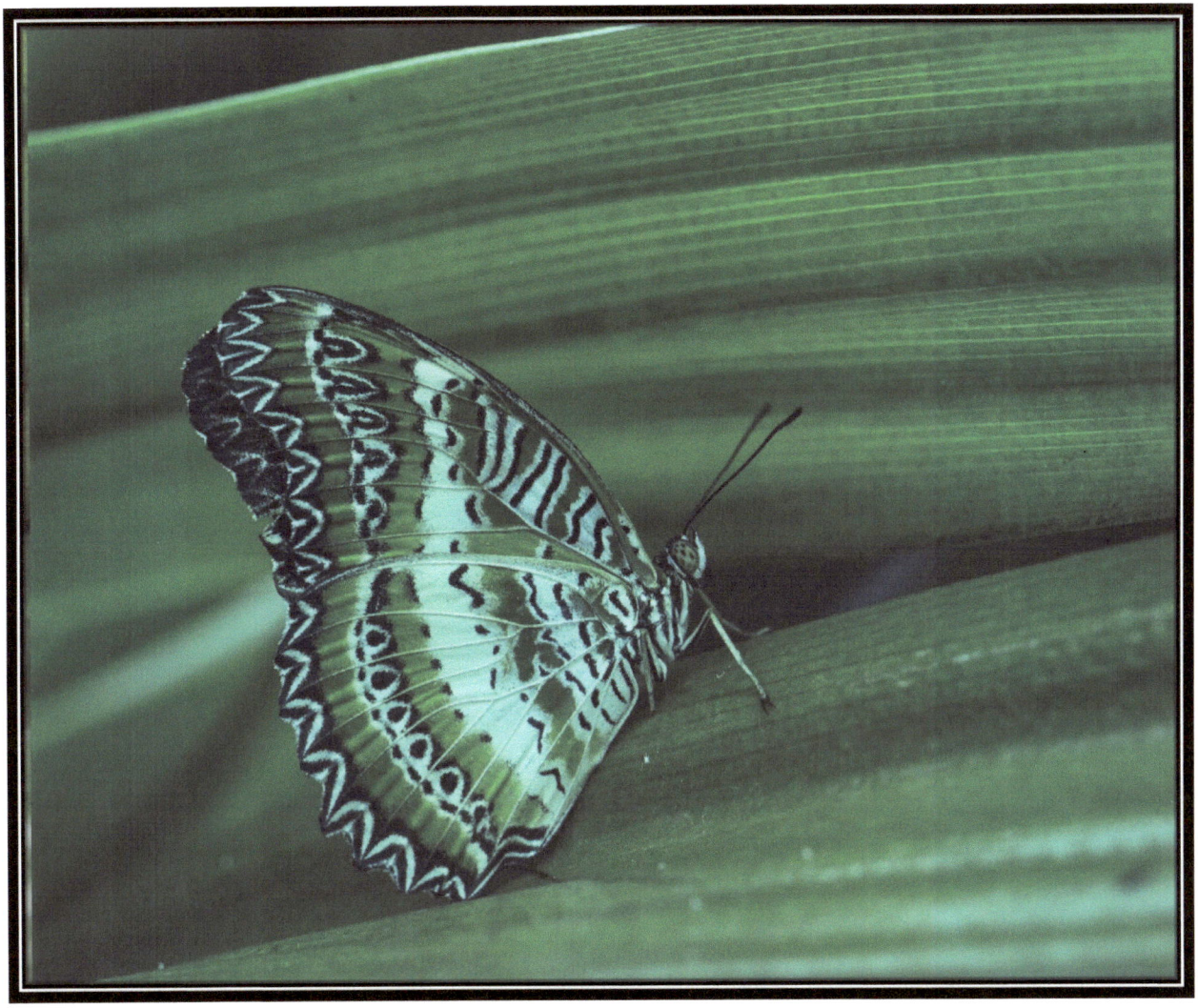

Image 3-3 Blanket Flower

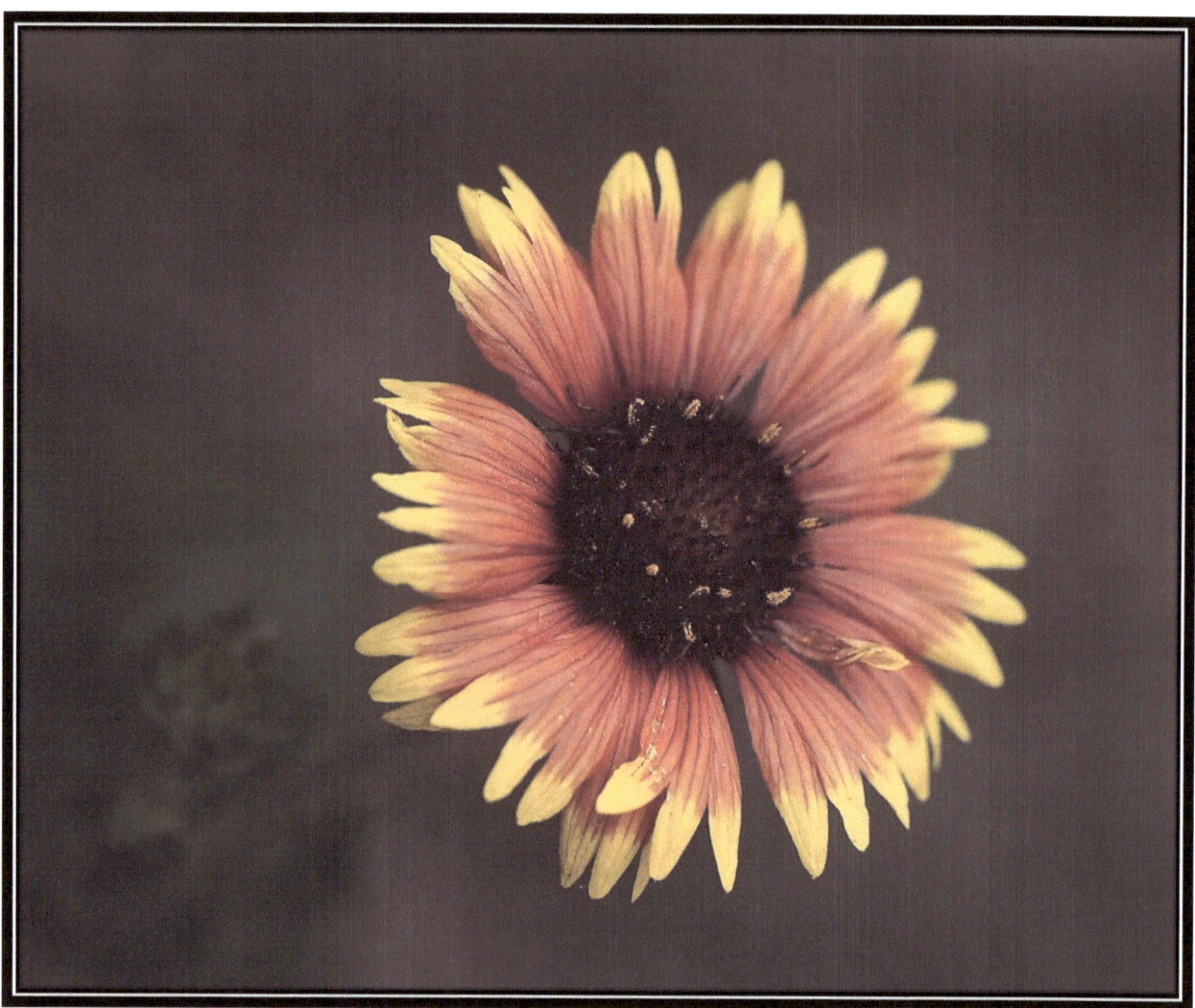

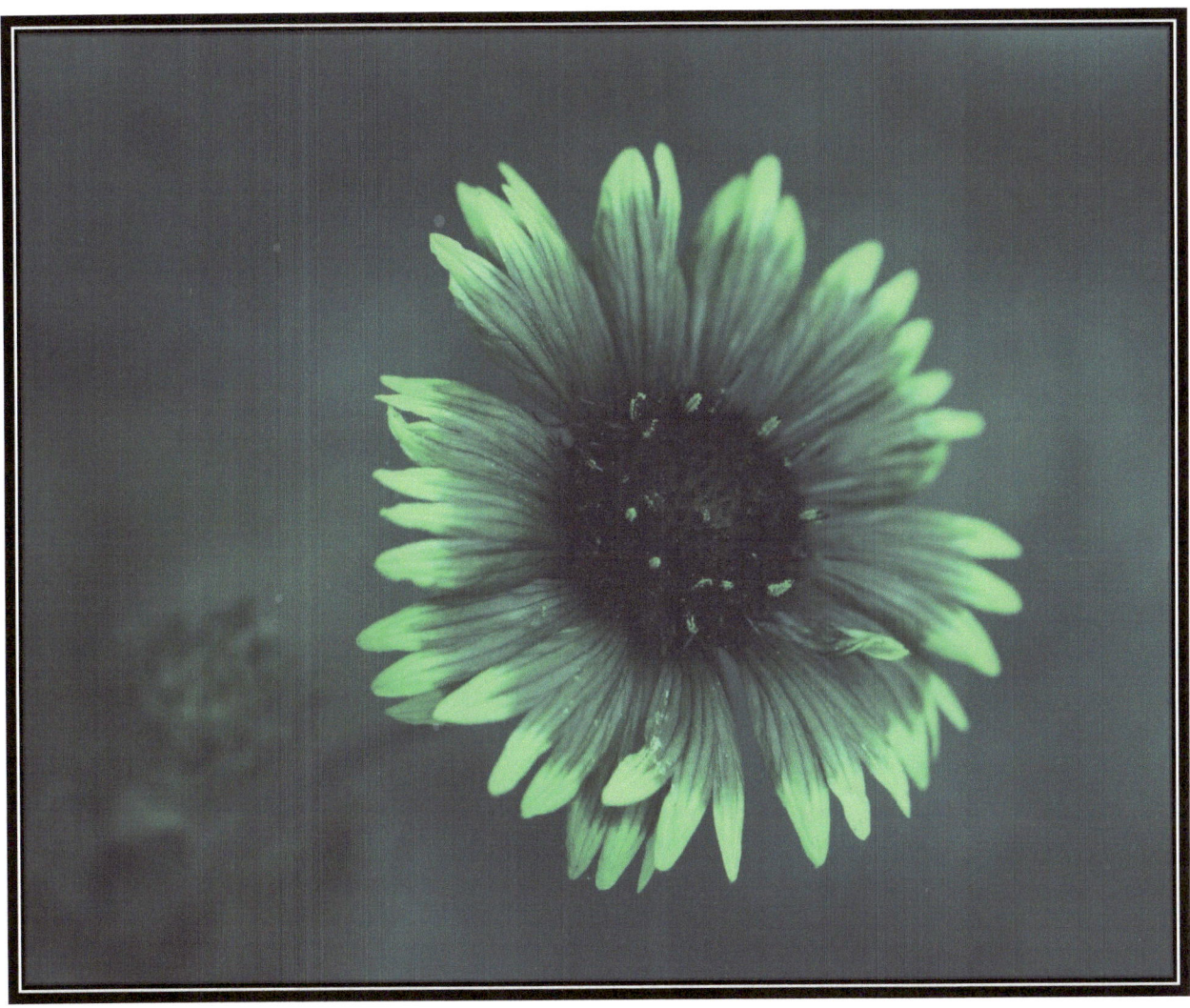

Image 3-4   Hibiscus

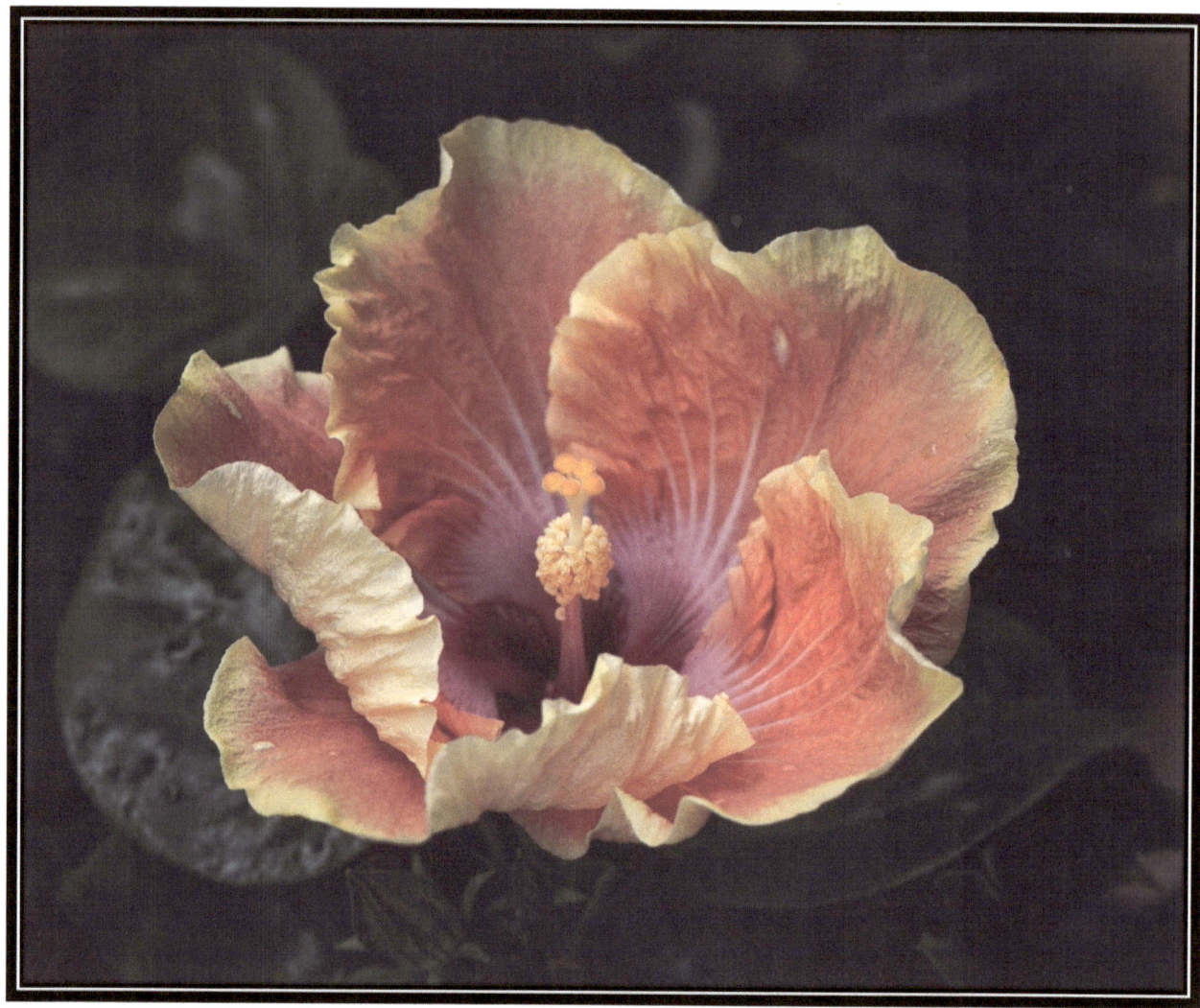

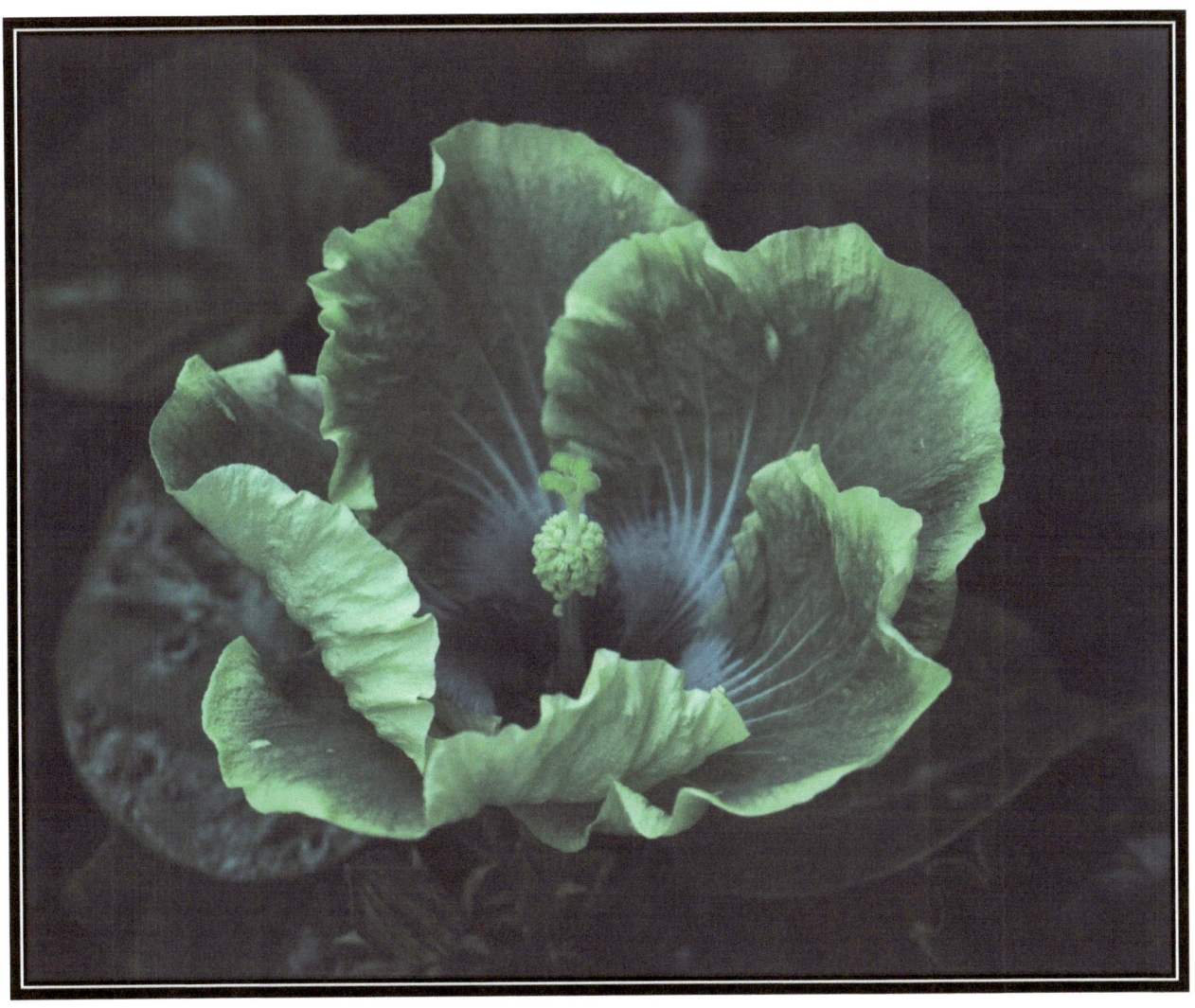

Image 3-5 Pomegranates

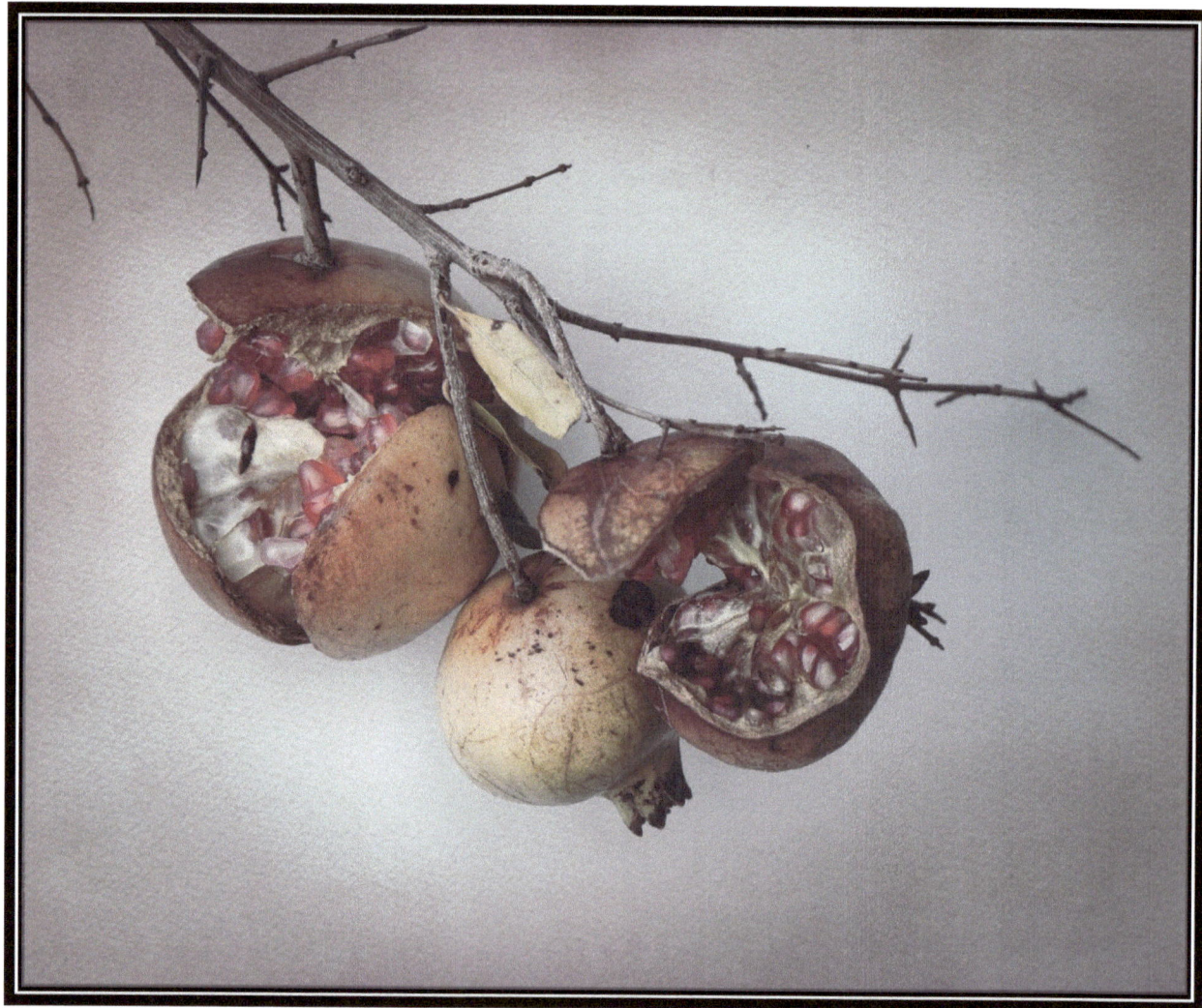

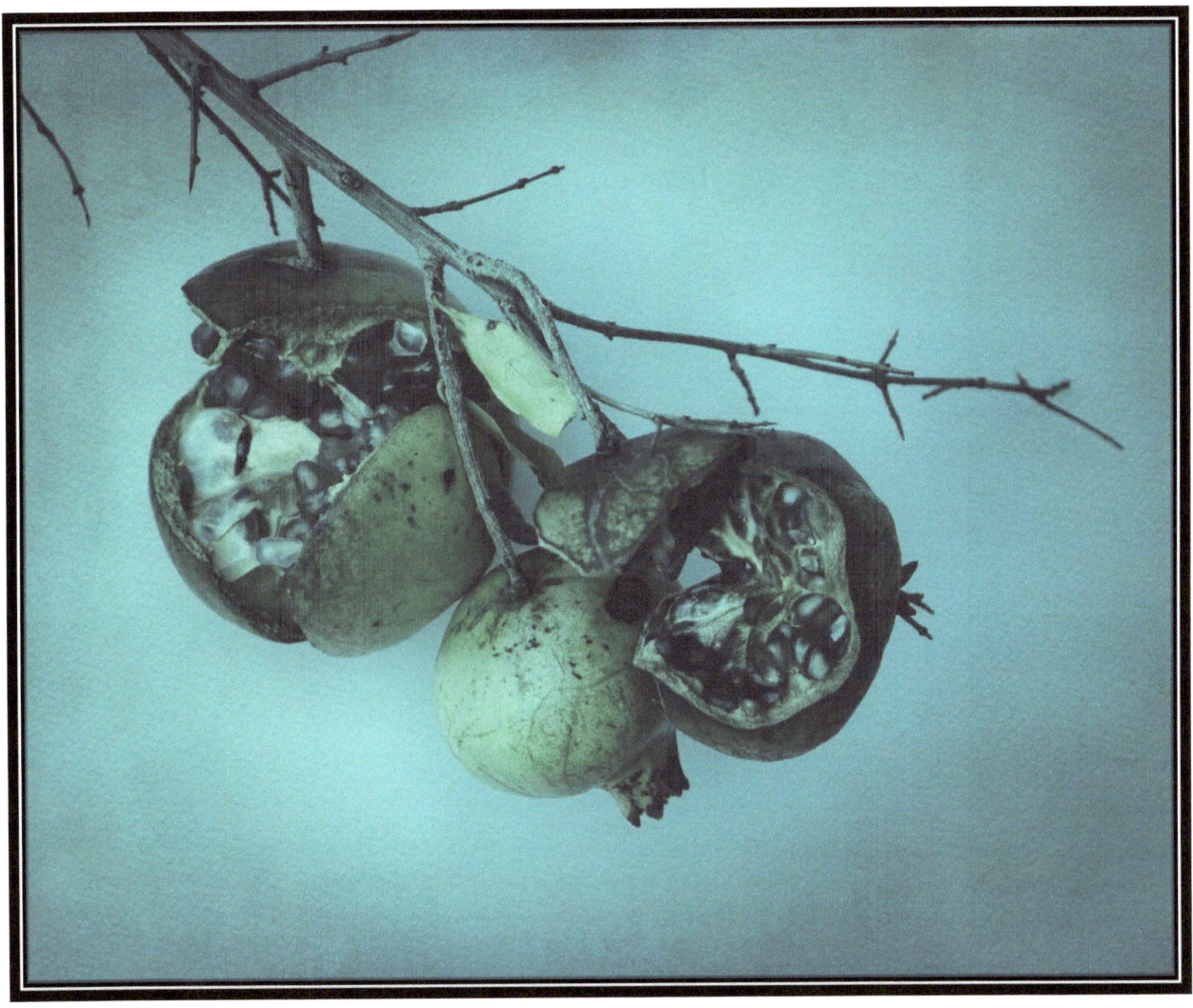

Image 3-6   "The Road Less Traveled"

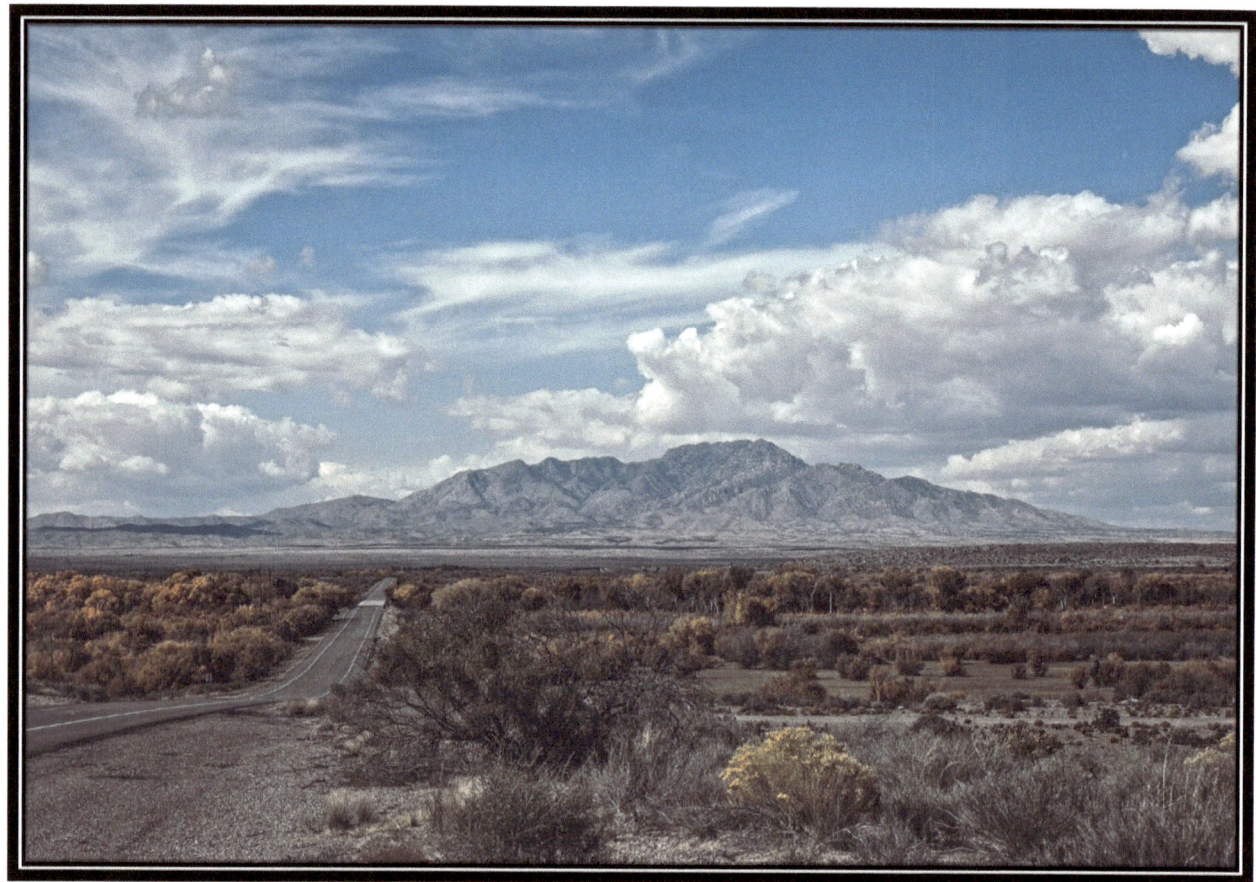

SEEING COLOR COLORBLIND

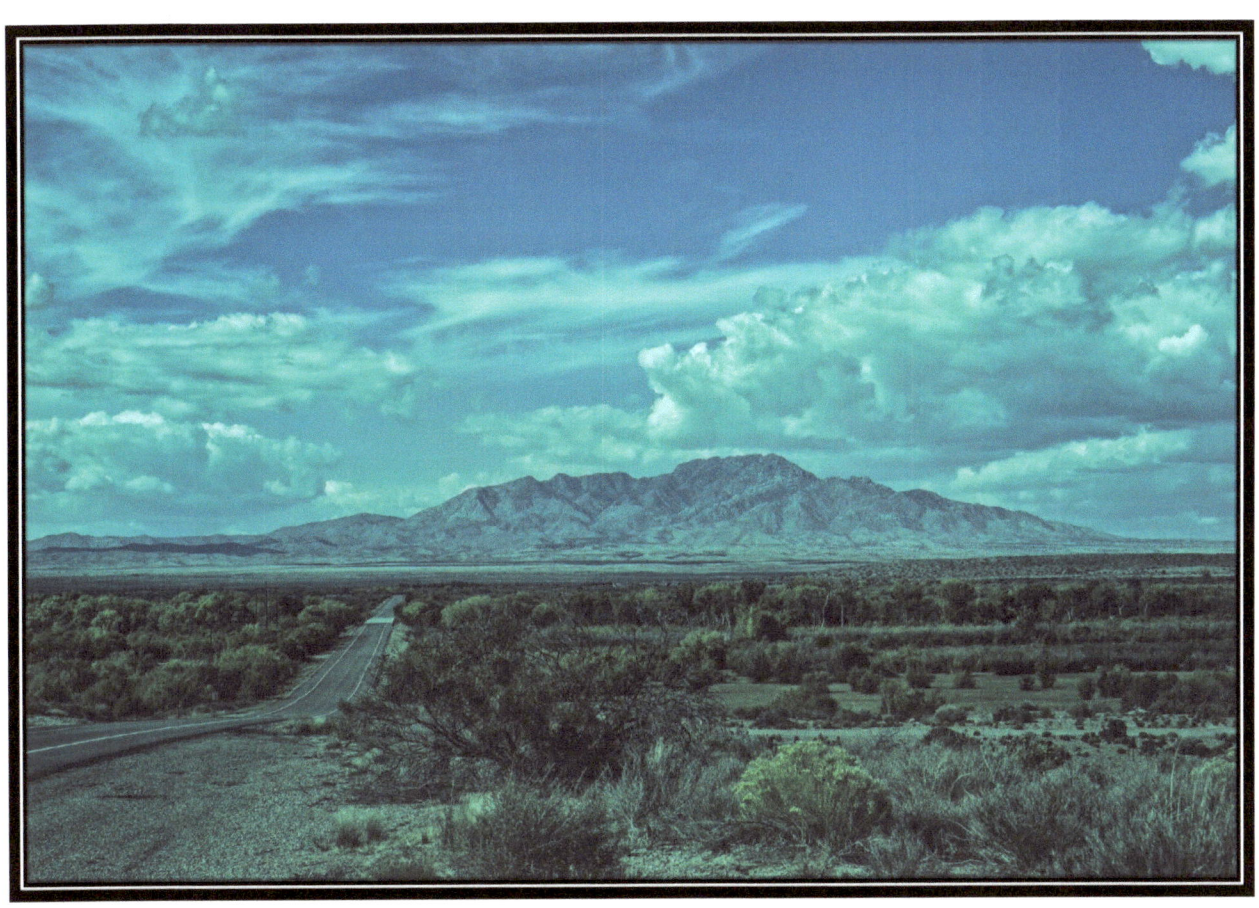

SUSAN BRANDT GRAHAM

4 YELLOWS

To the red dichromat, yellows vary from shades that I would call chartreuse to cyan. To me, the yellows as seen through red deficient eyes are beautiful in their own right.

Image 4-1   Wildflower

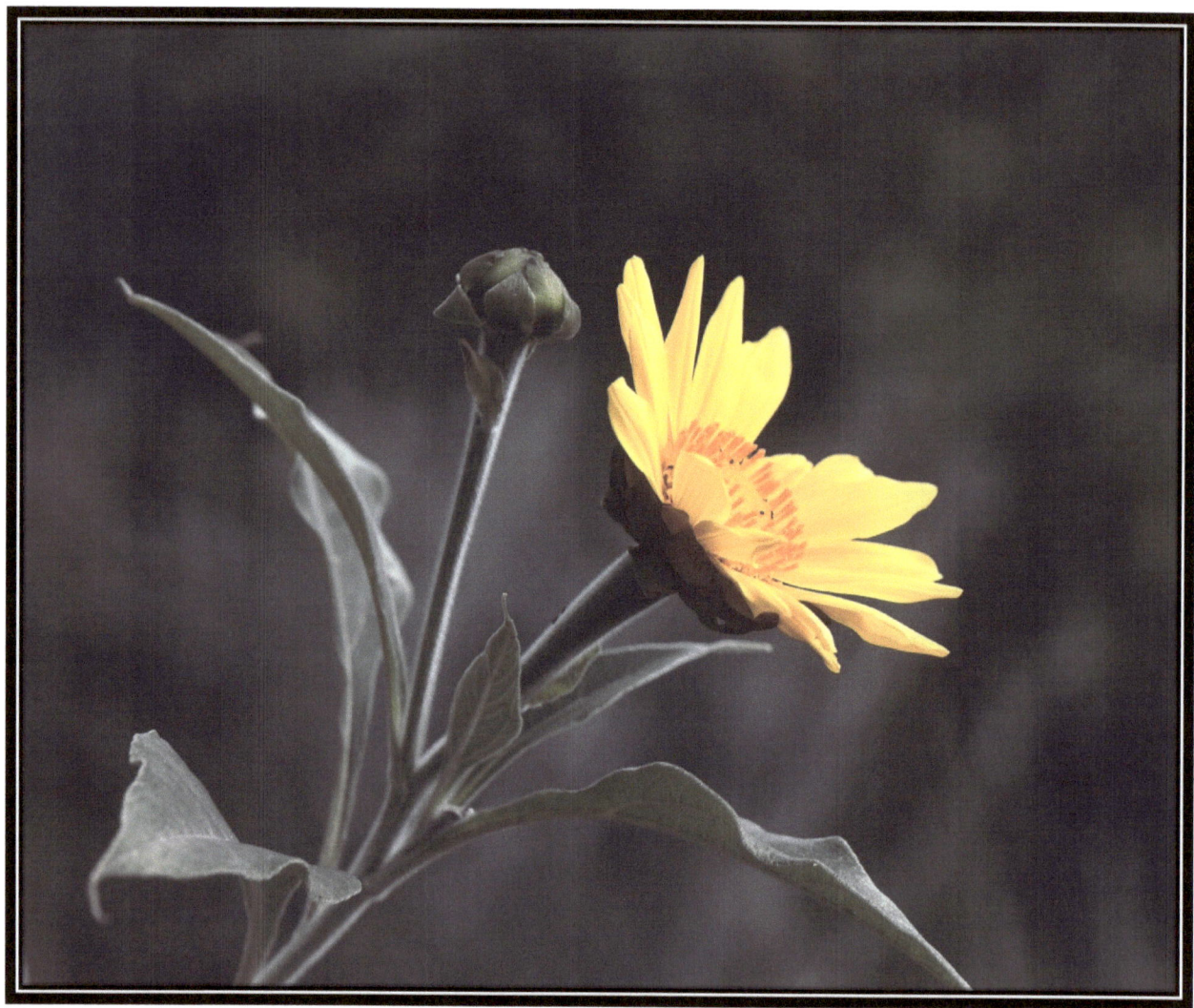

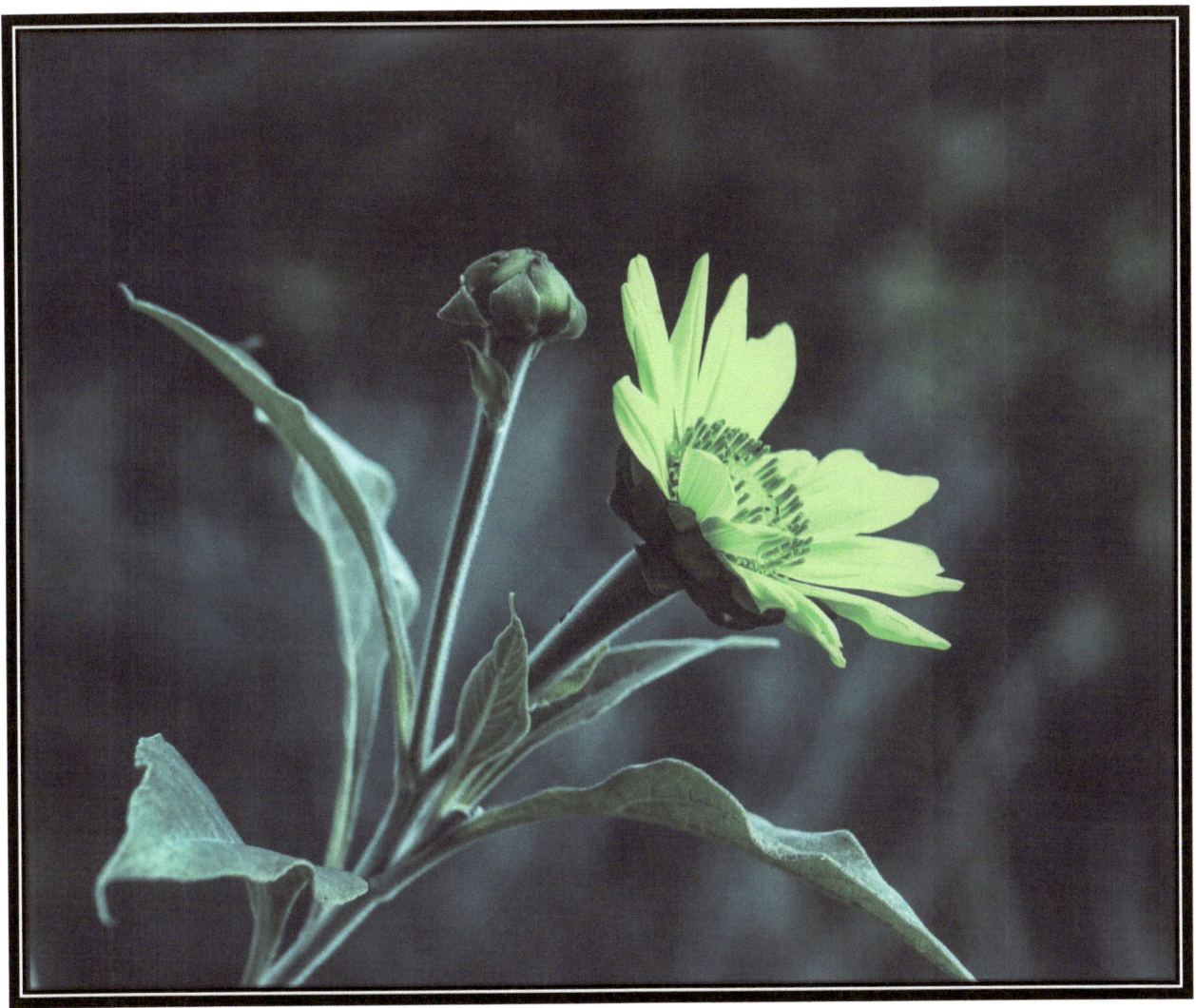

Image 4-2   Rose 'Gold Medal'

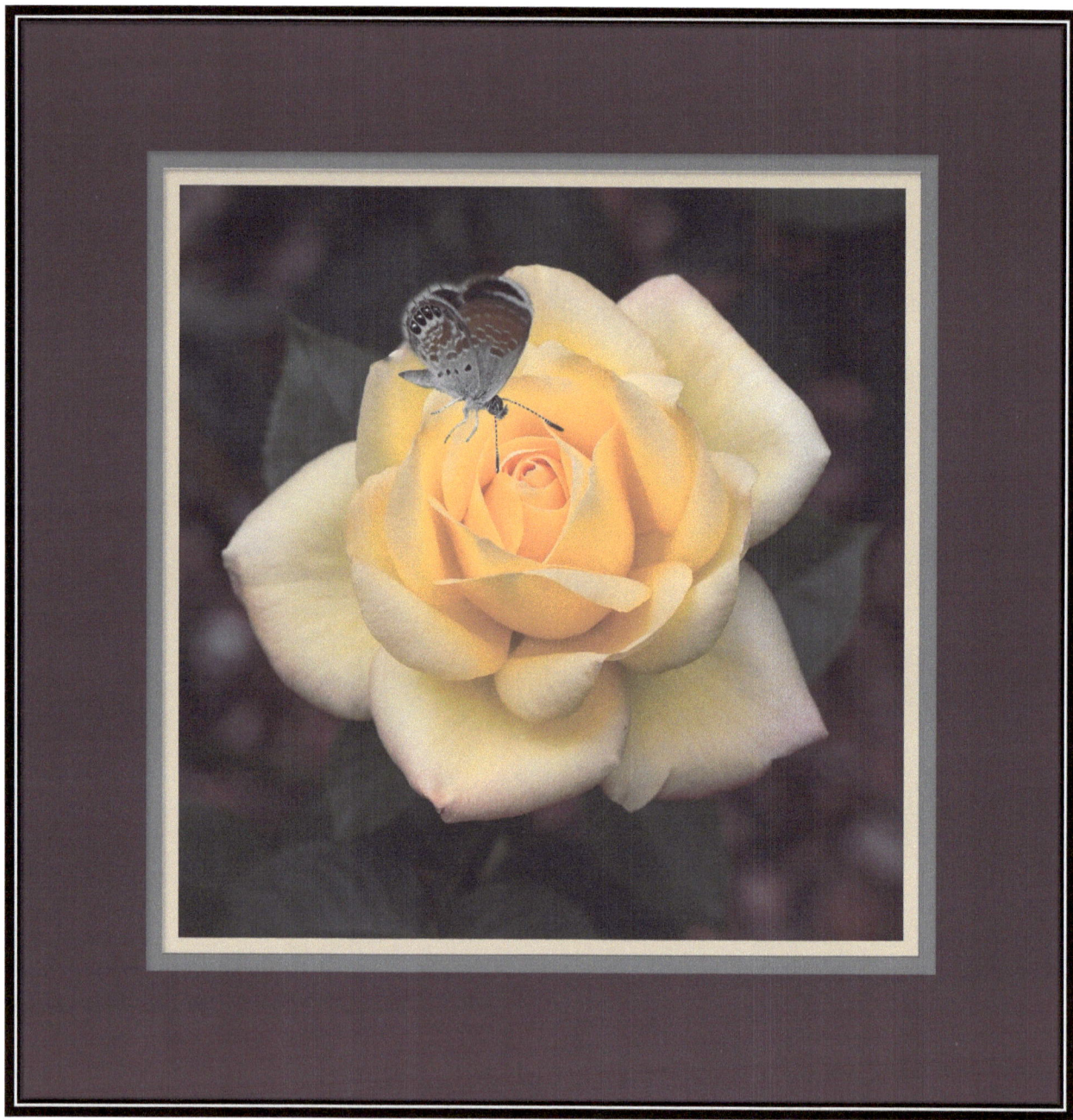

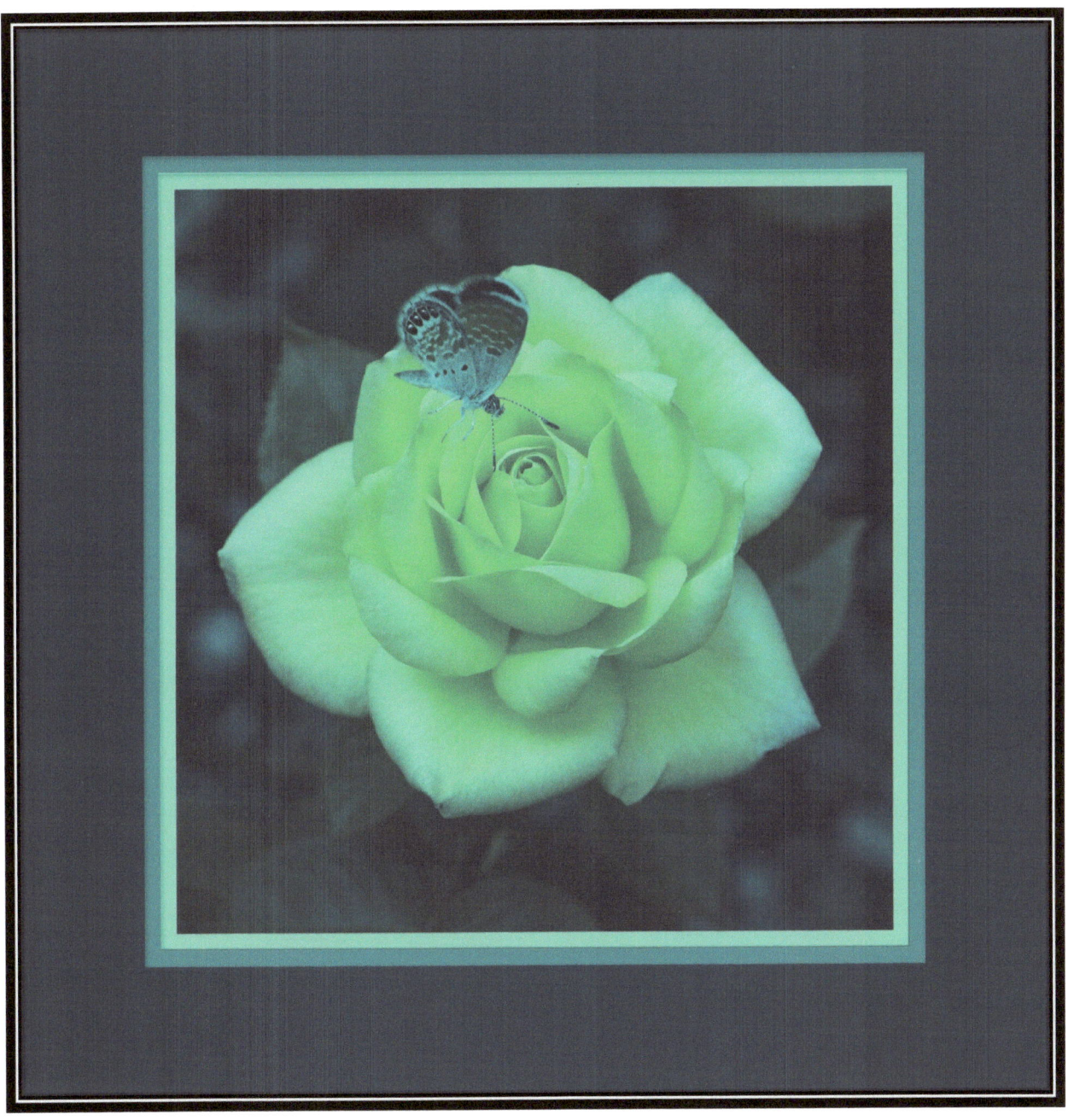

Image 4-3   African Iris

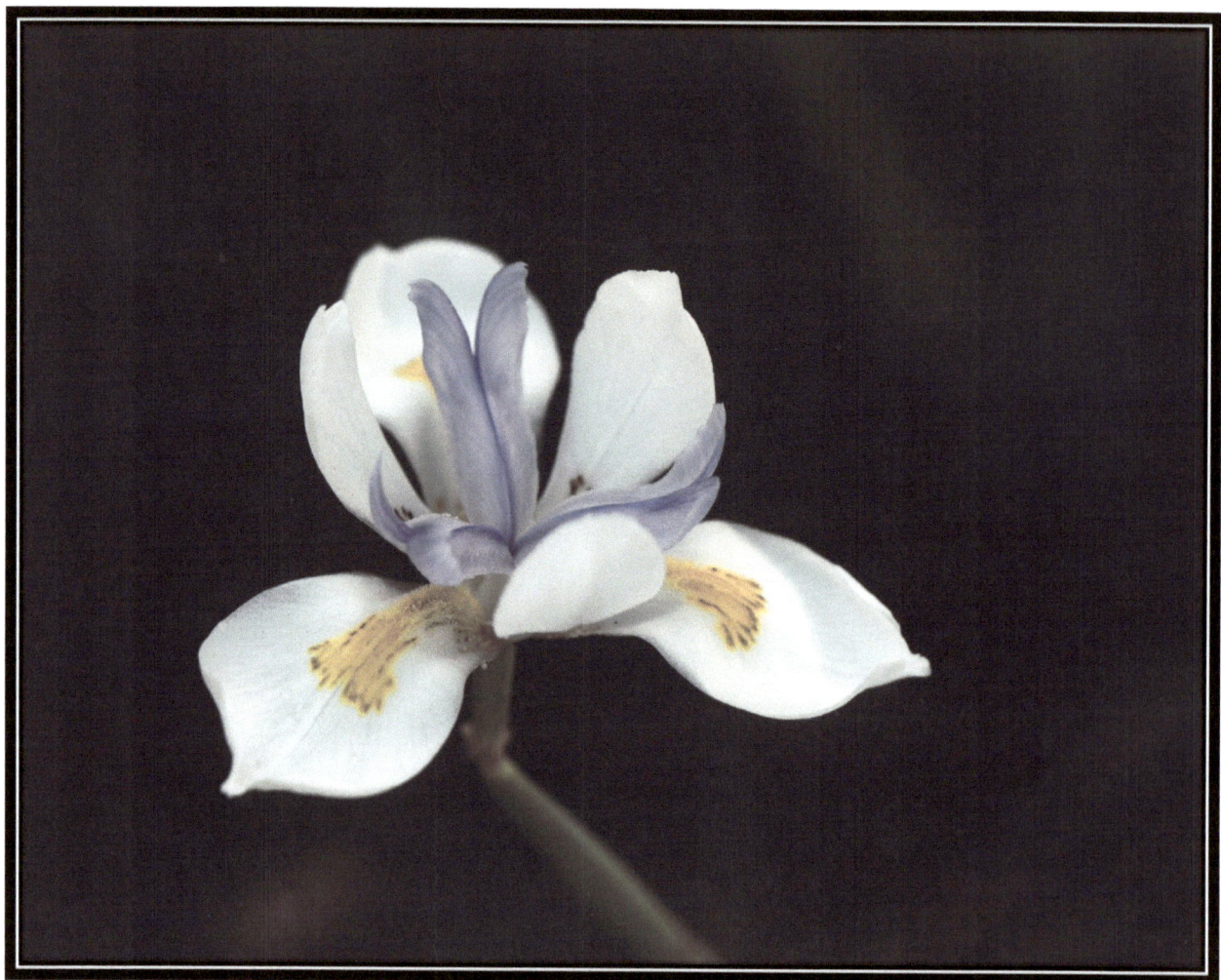

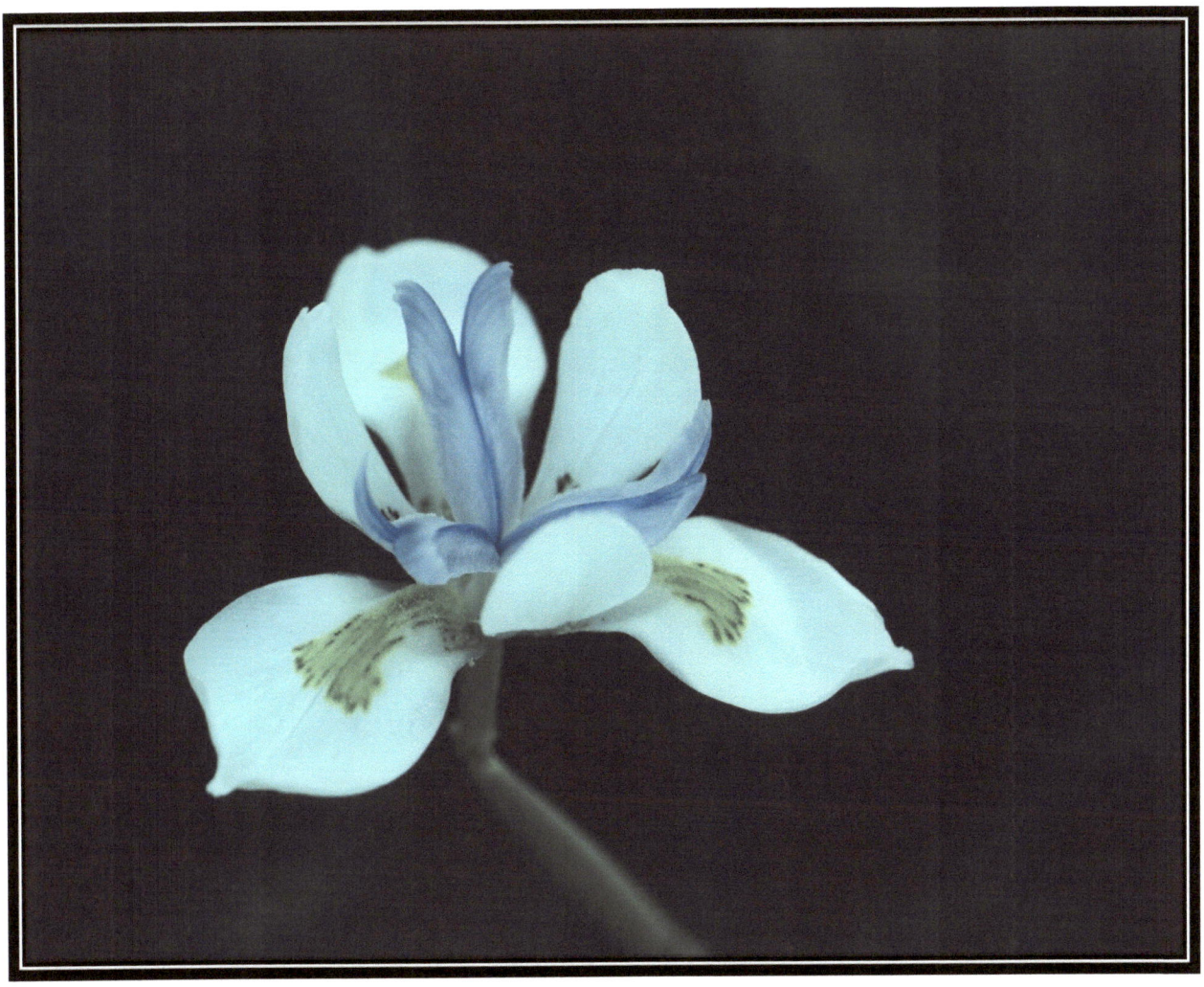

SUSAN BRANDT GRAHAM

5 BLUES

True blues are seen by the red dichromat as they are seen by people with normal color vision.

Image 5-1 "The Observer/The Observed"

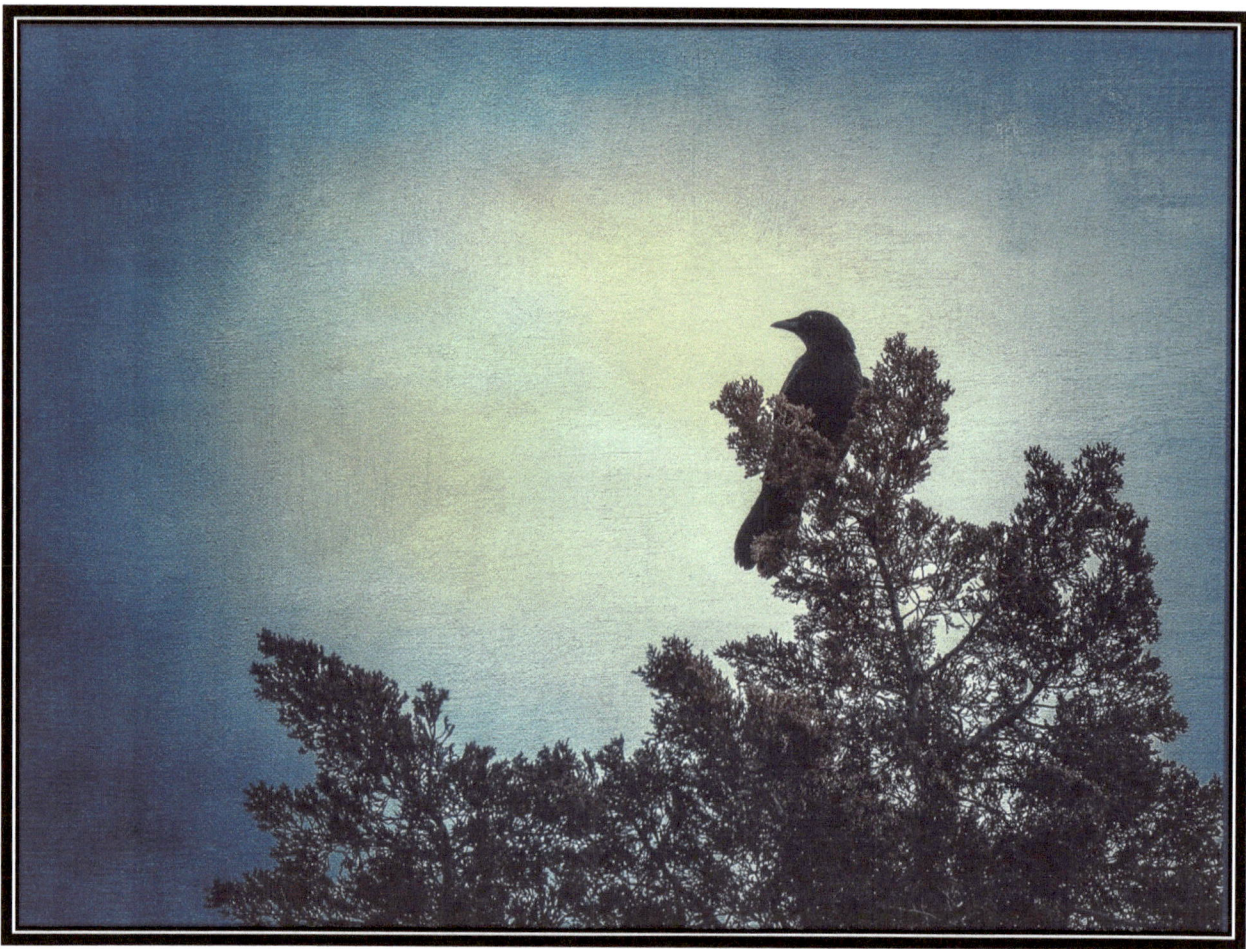

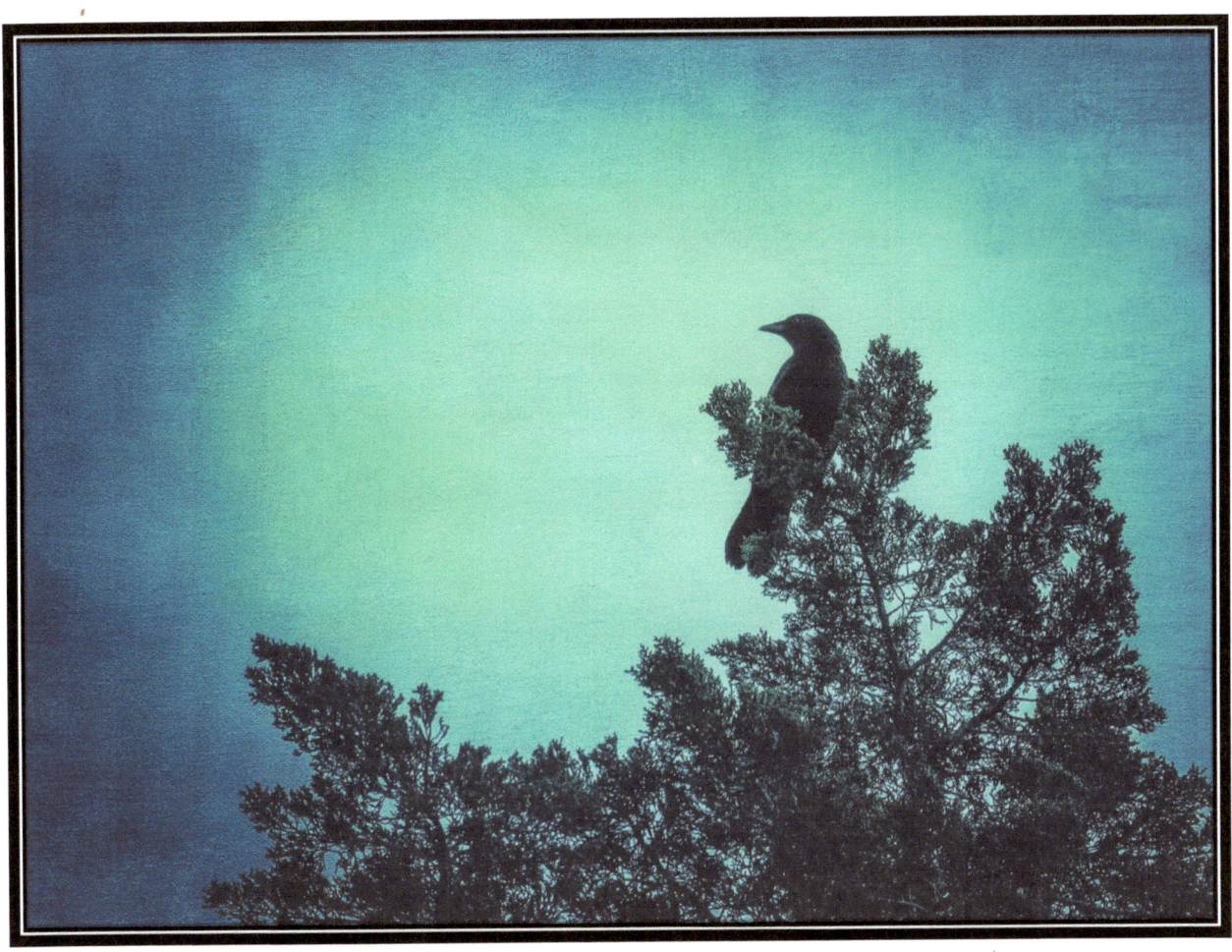

Image 5-2 "Monsoon Skies – Turmoil"

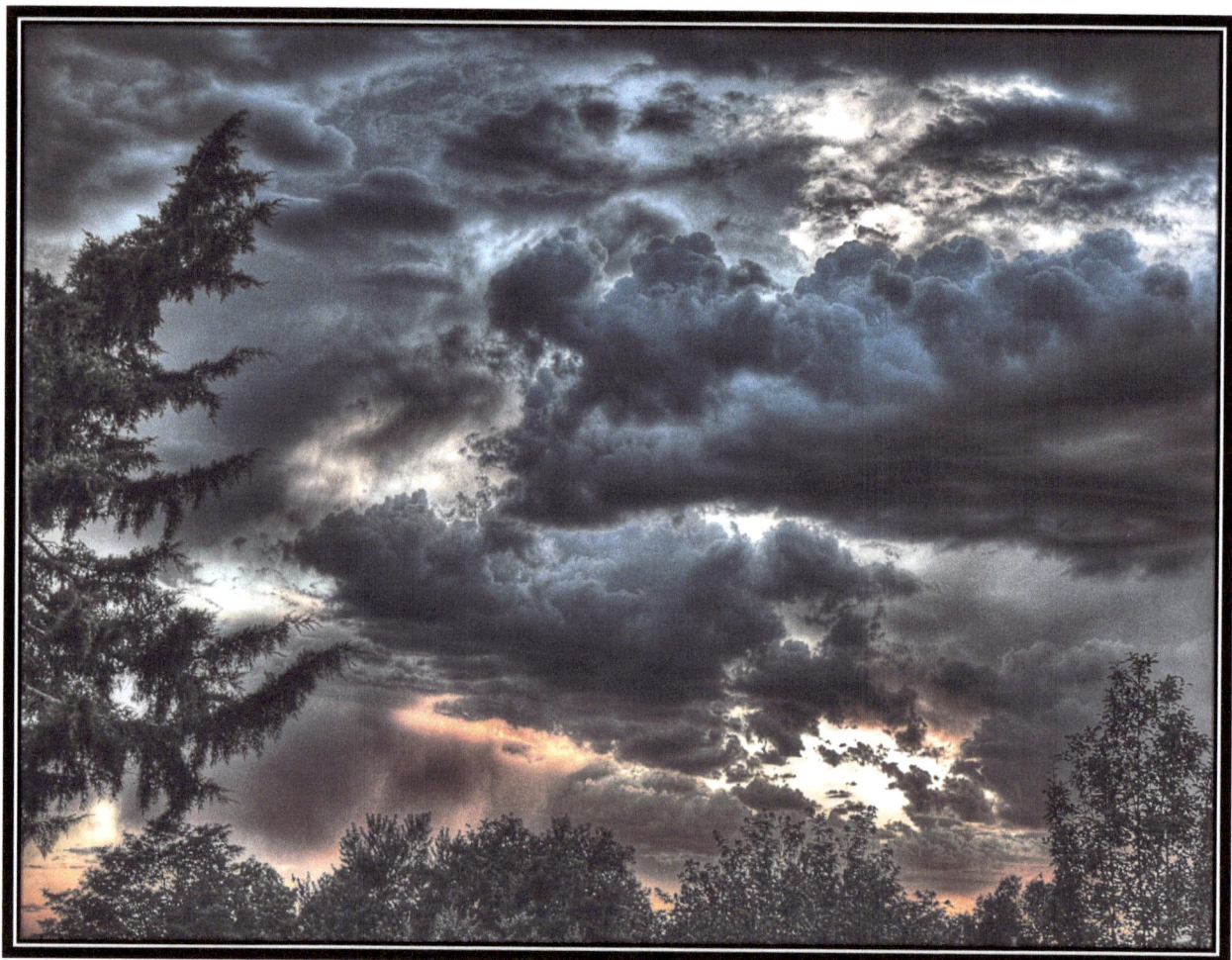

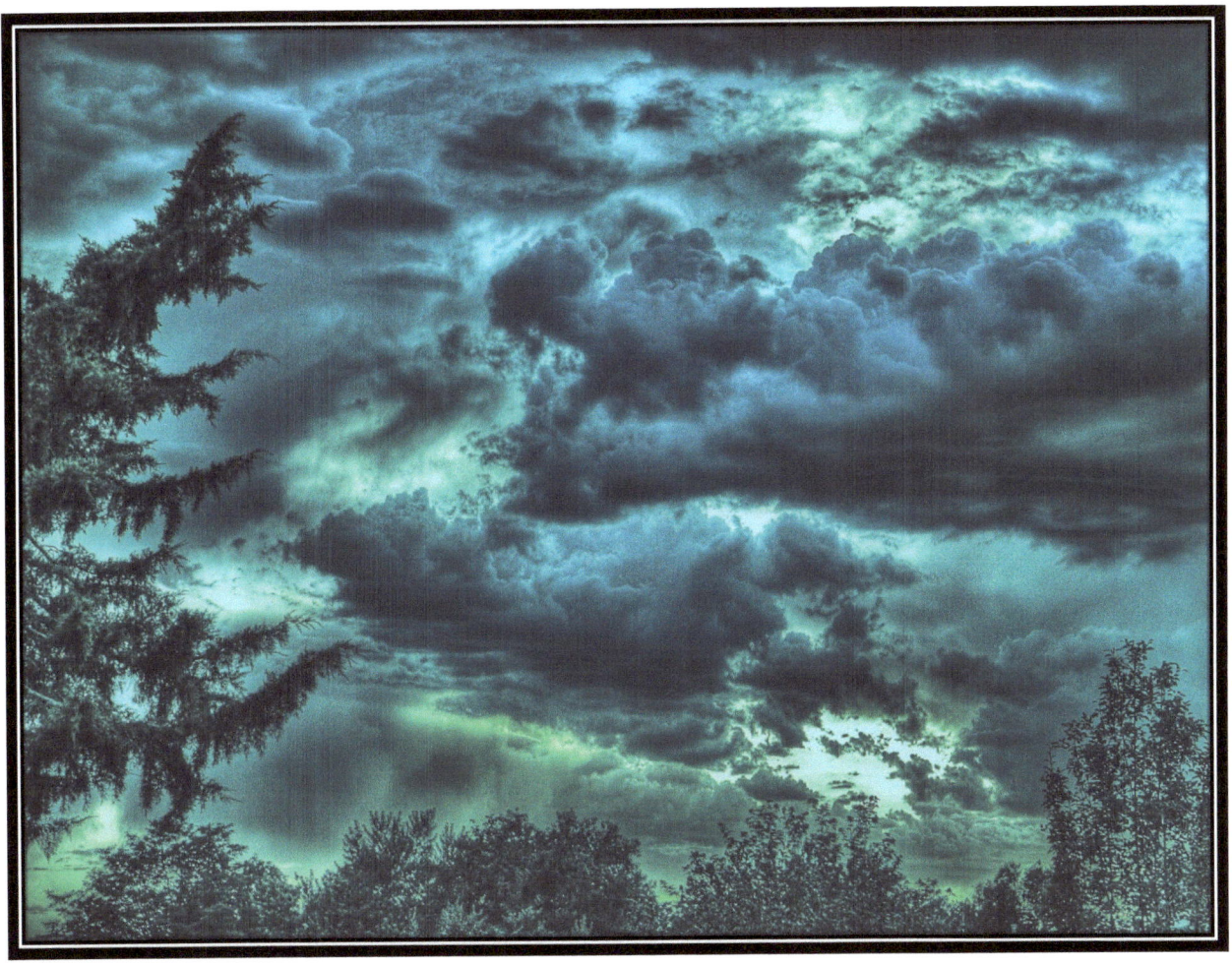

SUSAN BRANDT GRAHAM

6 MONOCHROME, AND BLACK AND WHITE

As in previous images, red in a monochromatic image is not seen by a red dichromat. The object will, instead, be perceived in some shade or shades of blue, green, and cyan.

Of all the pairs of diptychs in this series, the ones in black and white surprised me the most, initially; later skin tones became even more surprising. I had to ponder why all that cyan appeared in the black and white images. It was not unpleasant in appearance, just very strange to me.

In the RGB system, white light is made of all colors, while black is the absence of light. Pure white and pure grays contain equal amounts of red, green, and blue. If the cones of eye cannot perceive red light, even black and white images will appear in shades of green, blue, and their combination, cyan.

After all these years, I finally understood how my father and son, both severely red deficient, could see color on a black and white television. That had been a huge mystery in my life. Mystery solved...

Image 6-1   Bishop's Cap

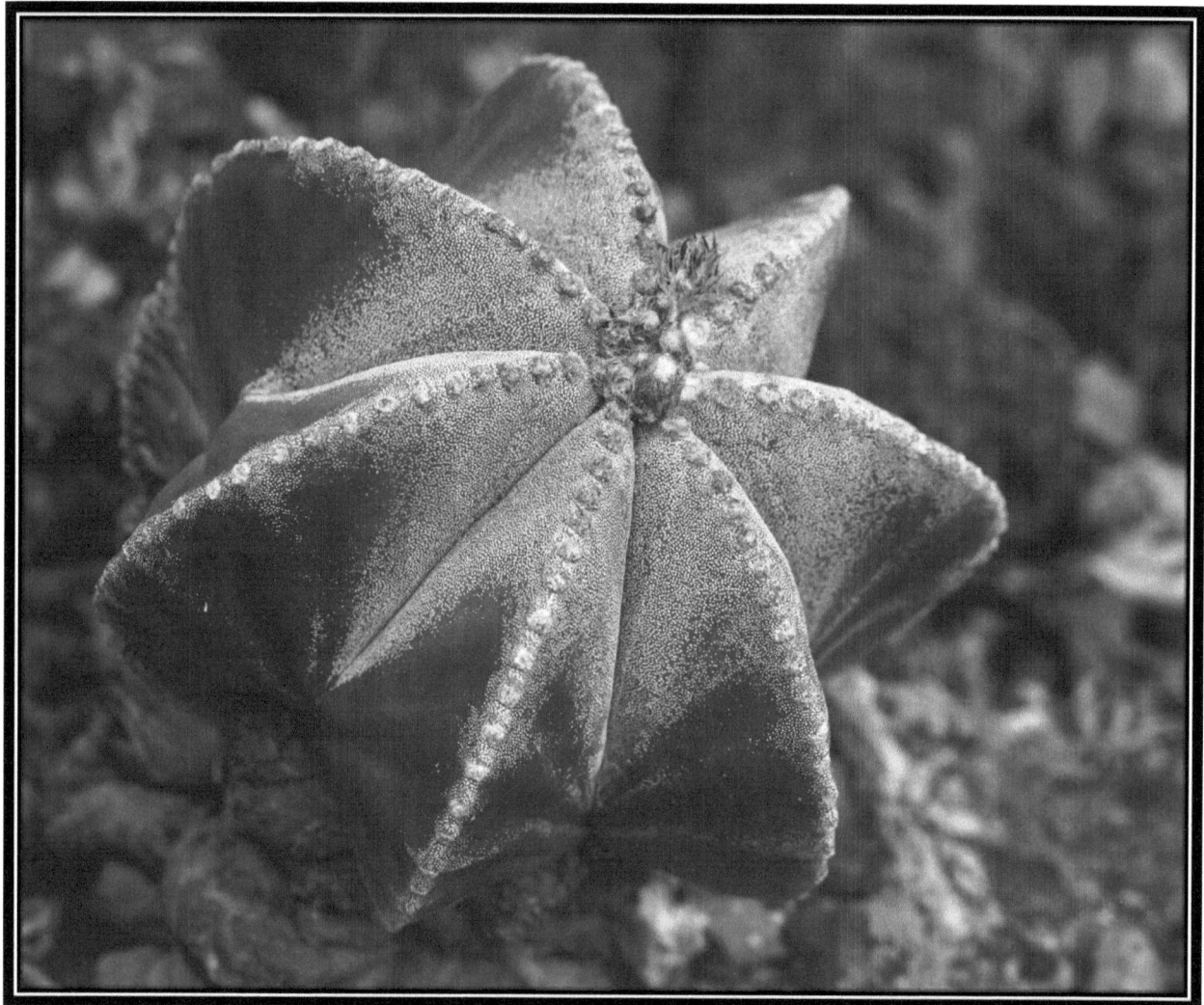

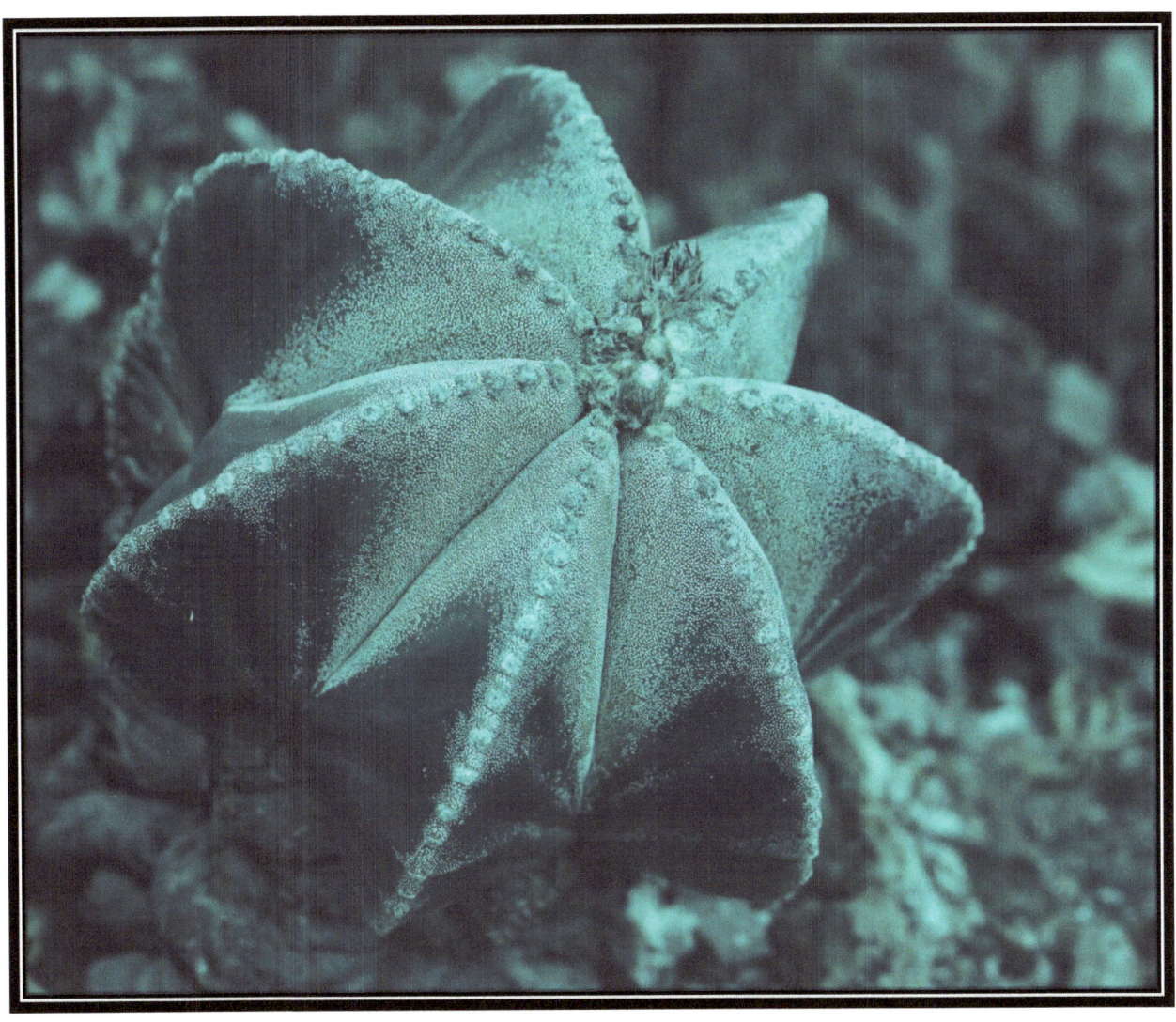

Image 6-2 Developing Pears

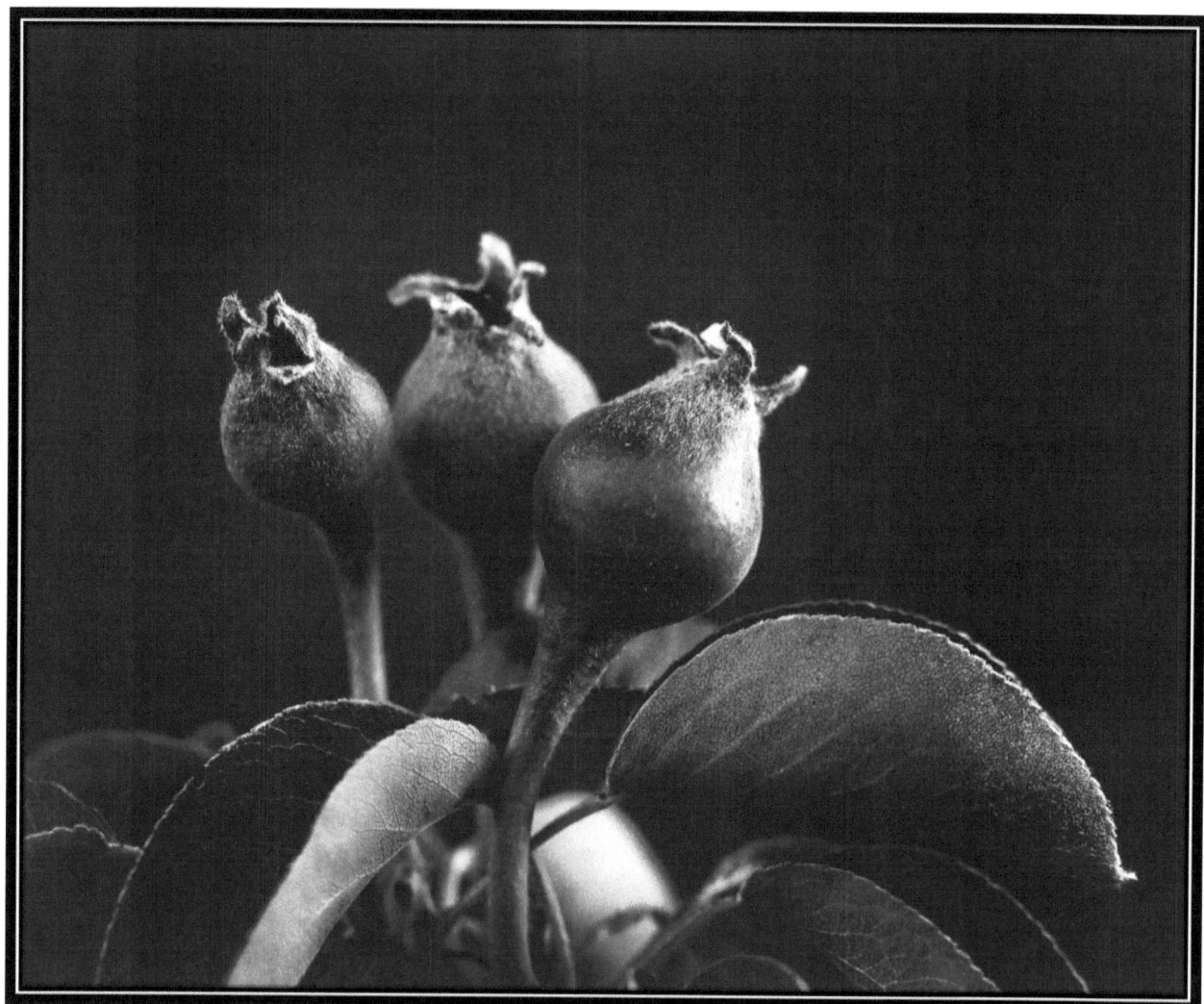

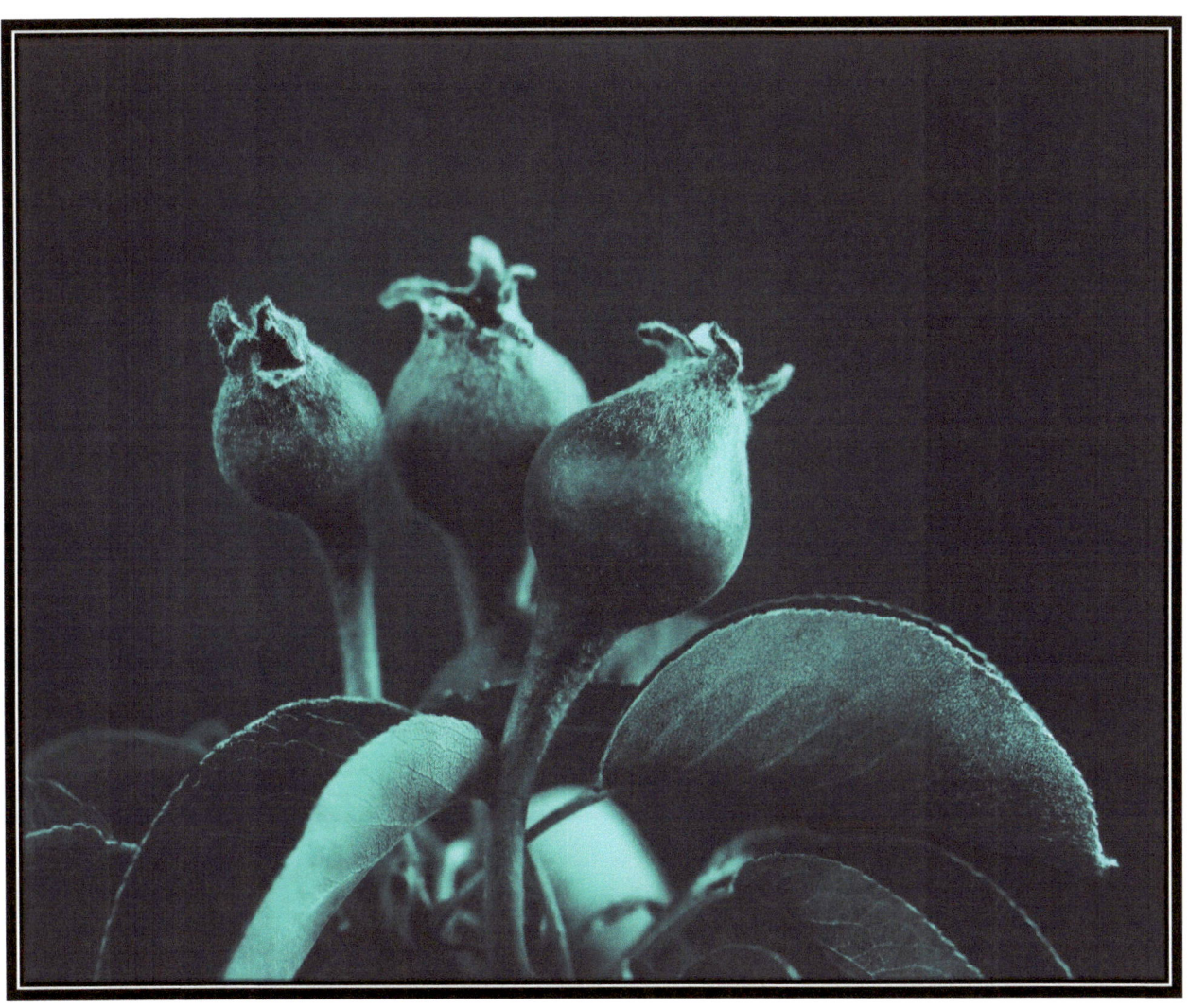

Image 6-3   Sunflower

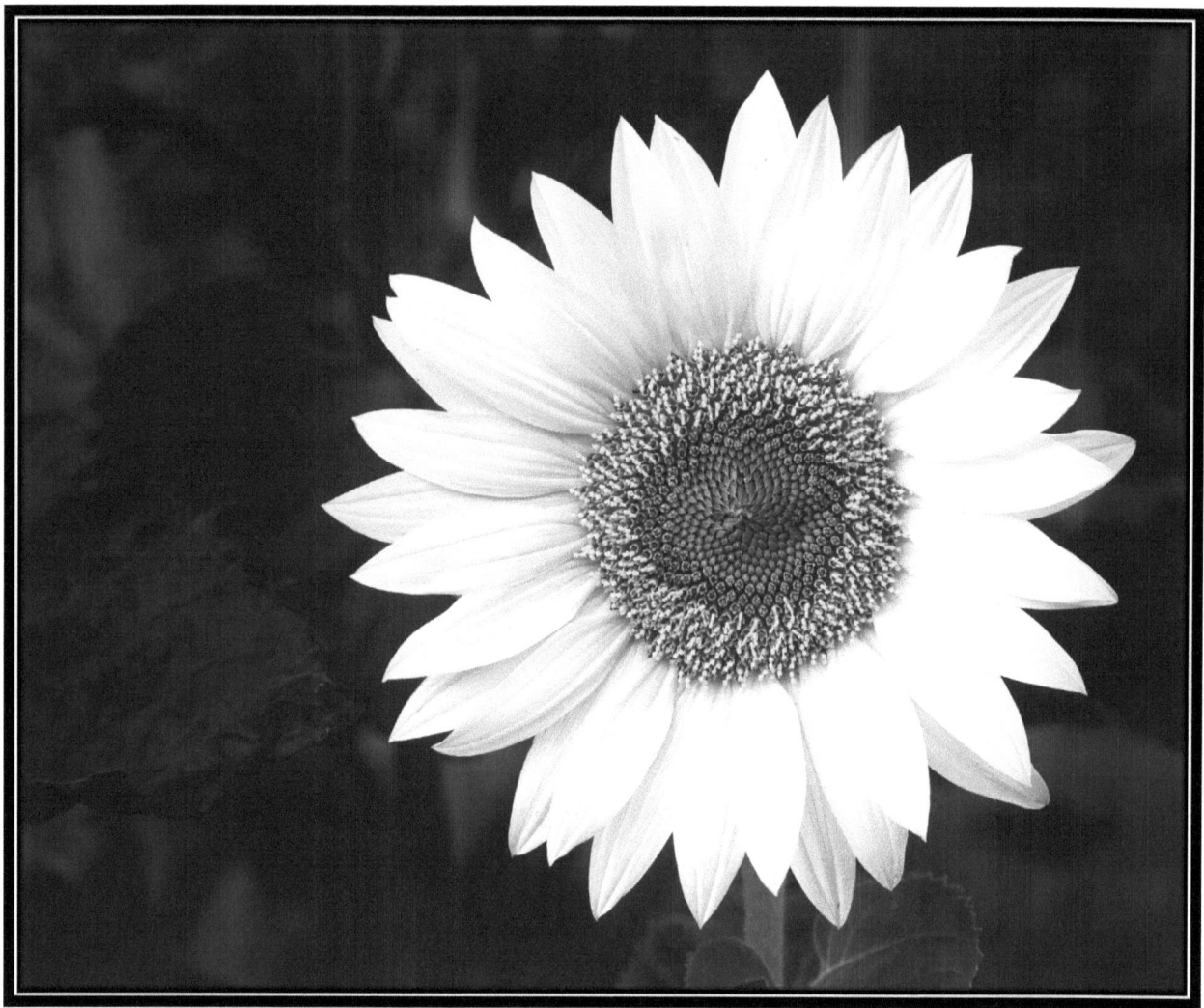

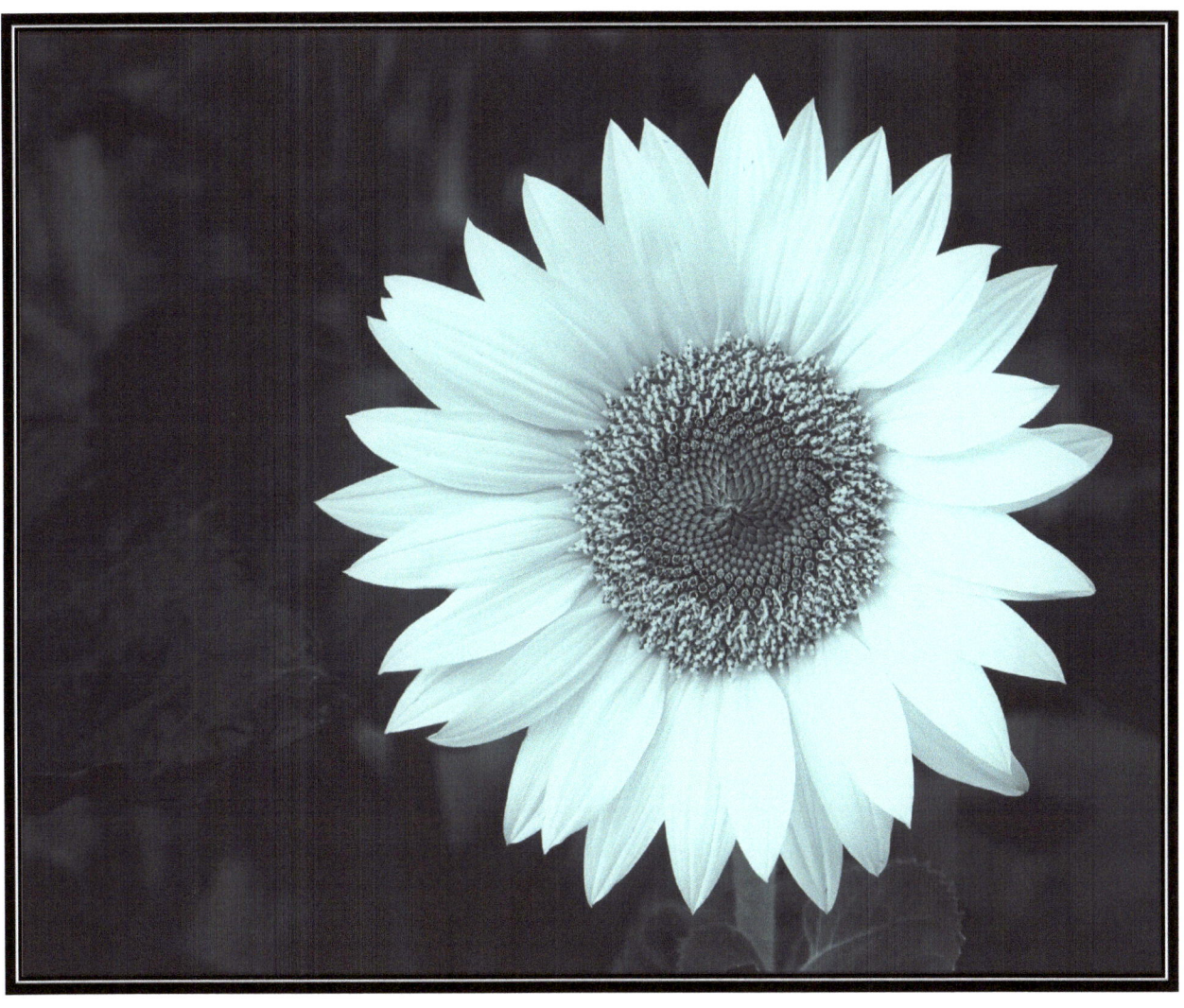

Image 6-4 Rose "Leonidas"

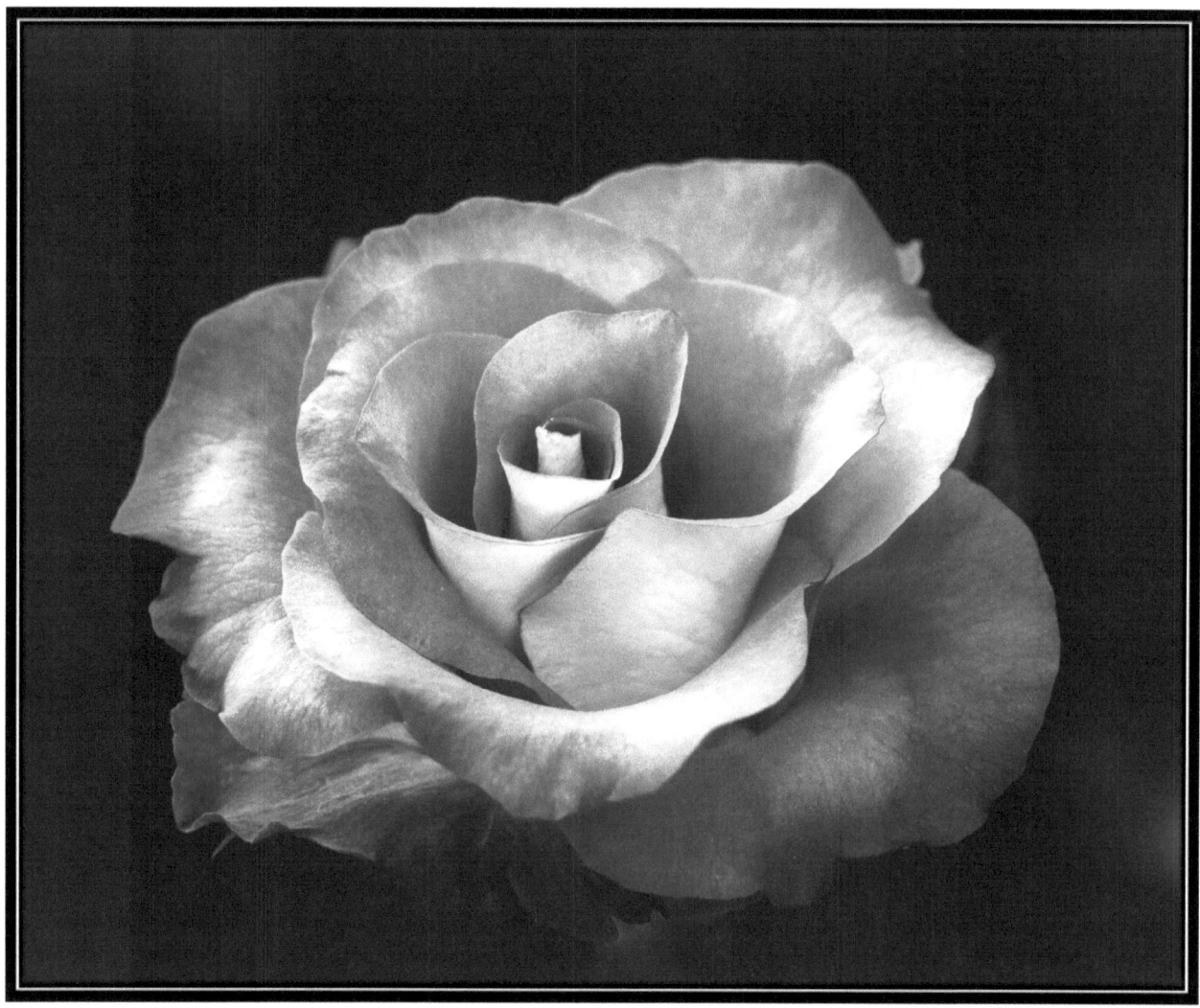

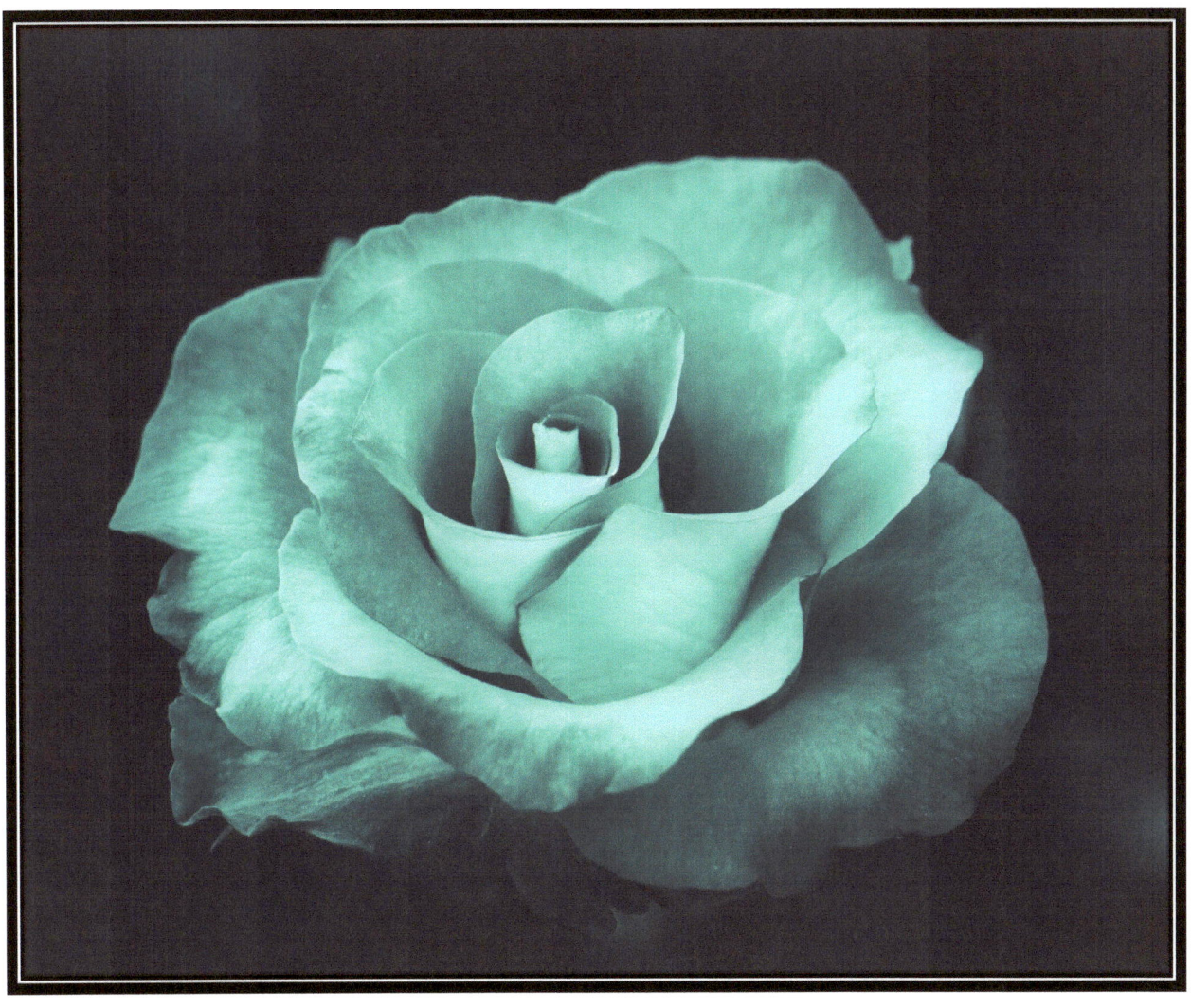

7 SKIN TONES

    Skin tones were probably the biggest surprise of all when I began to work on the diptychs comparing images seen by a person with normal color vision and by a person with severe red deficiency. It was the first time I realized my son saw me in various shades of cyan! I love wearing red lipstick, but when my son comes to visit I plan to wear lighter shades, which, hopefully, won't make me look so dead.

    The last two images in this section, "By My Choice" and "Turn, Turn, Turn," come from the series, "Persephone's Choice: Every Woman's Dilemma," available as an e-book at Amazon (http://amzn.com/B01AX1OAZG). The moon images in "Turn, Turn, Turn" are from the Blood Red Total Lunar Eclipse of September 27, 2015, as photographed by me in New Mexico. When I saw the conversion, I understood why my son said he saw nothing special to stay up watching, while for me it was one of the more amazing celestial events of my lifetime.

Image 7-1   Mother

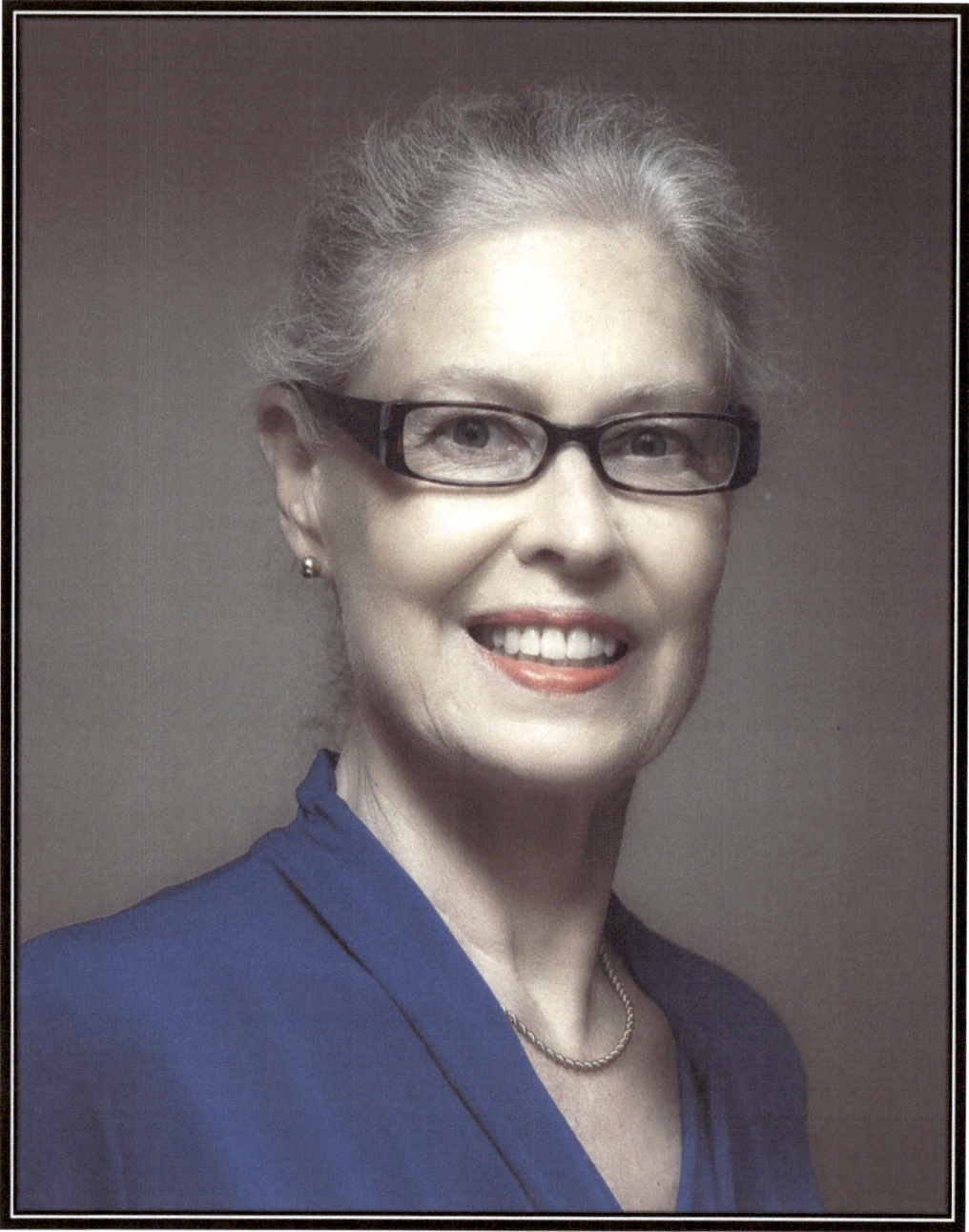

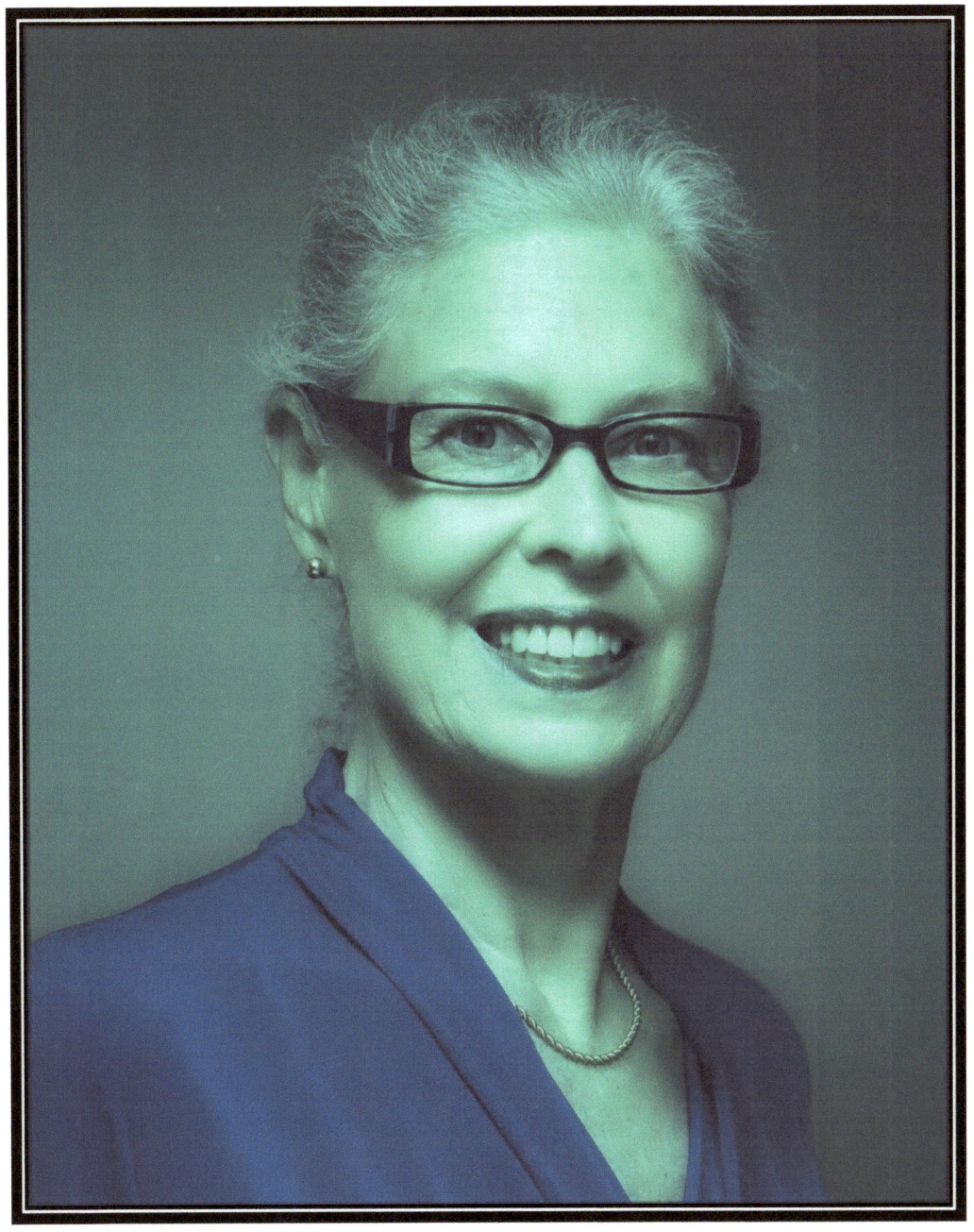

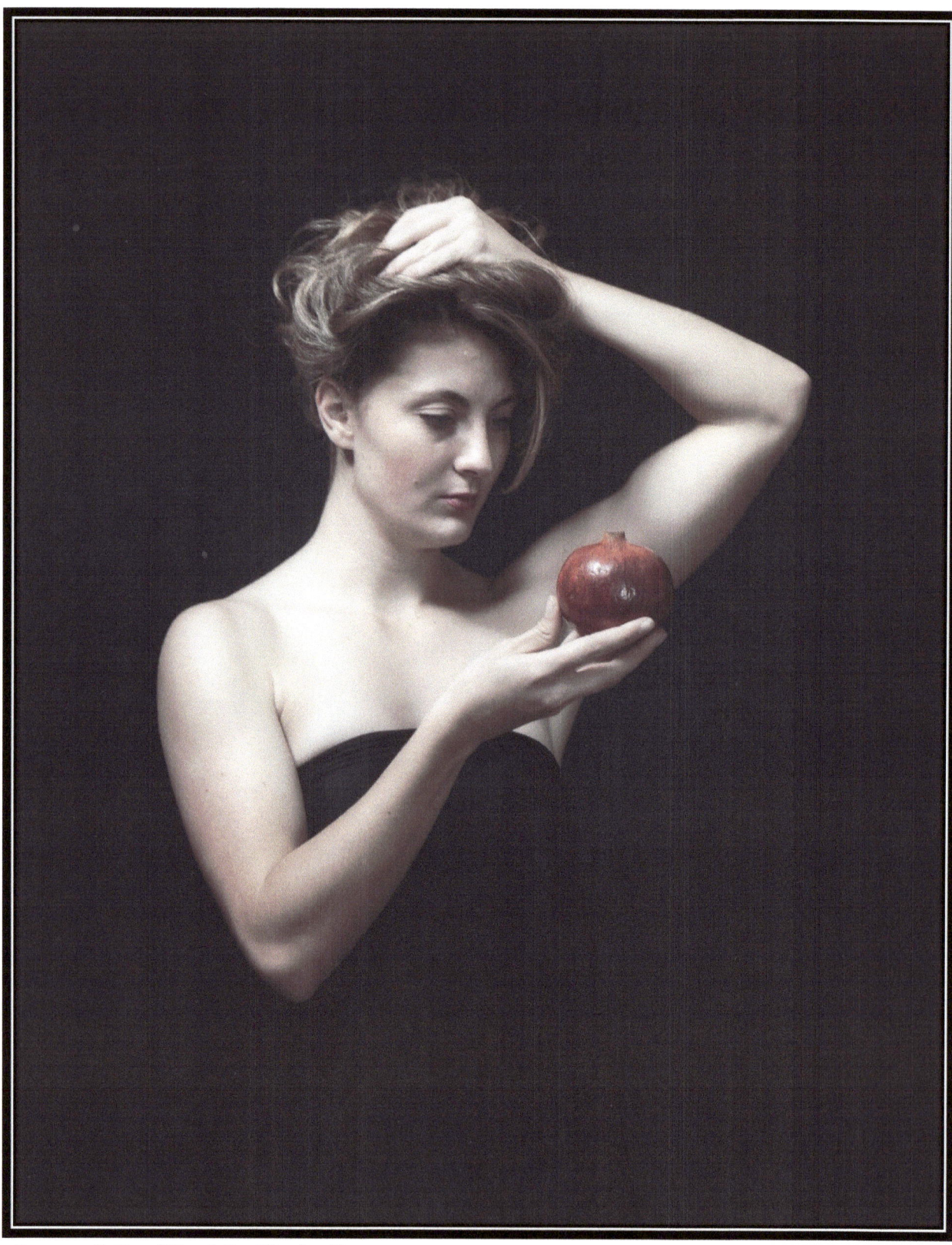

Image 7-2 "By My Choice"

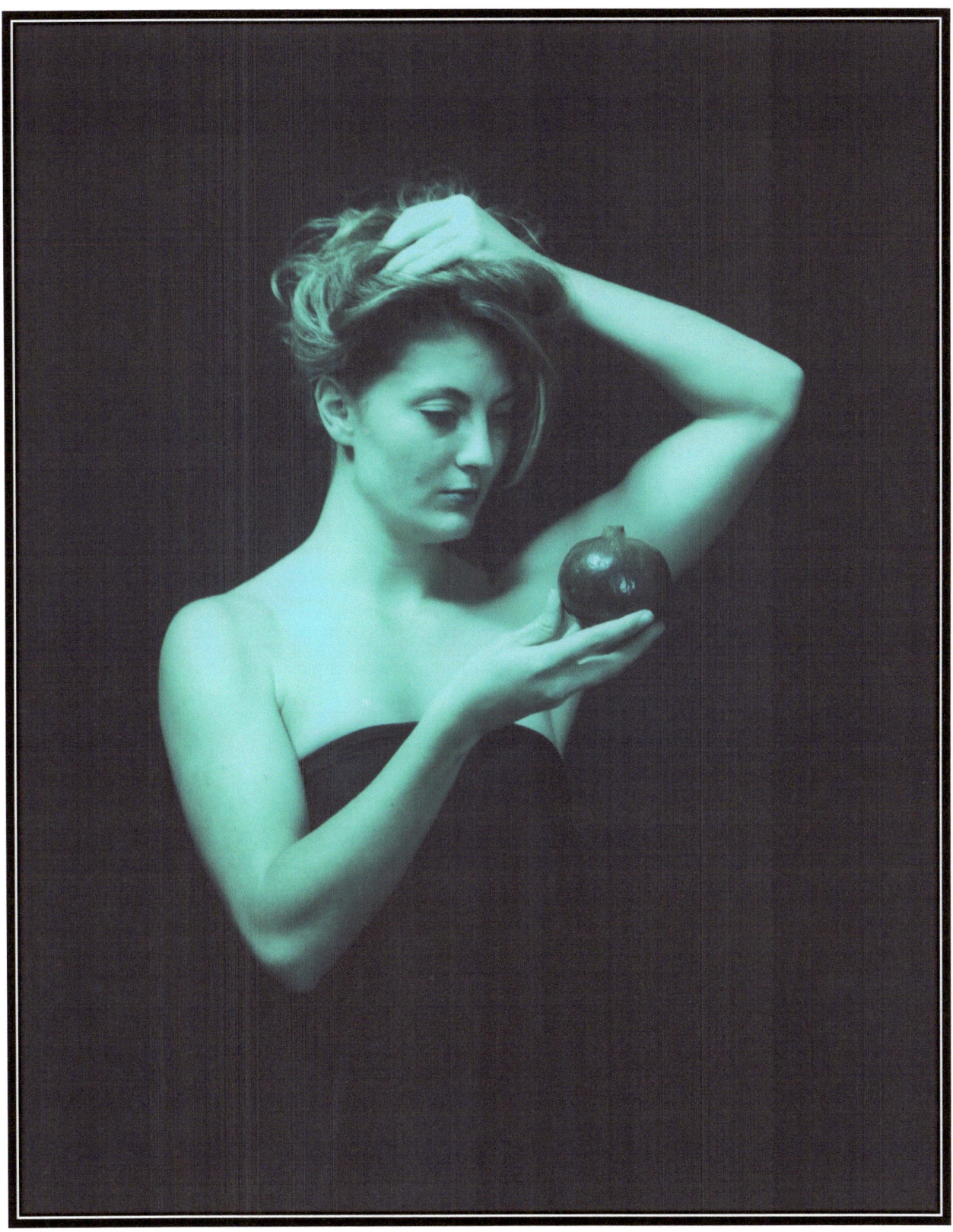

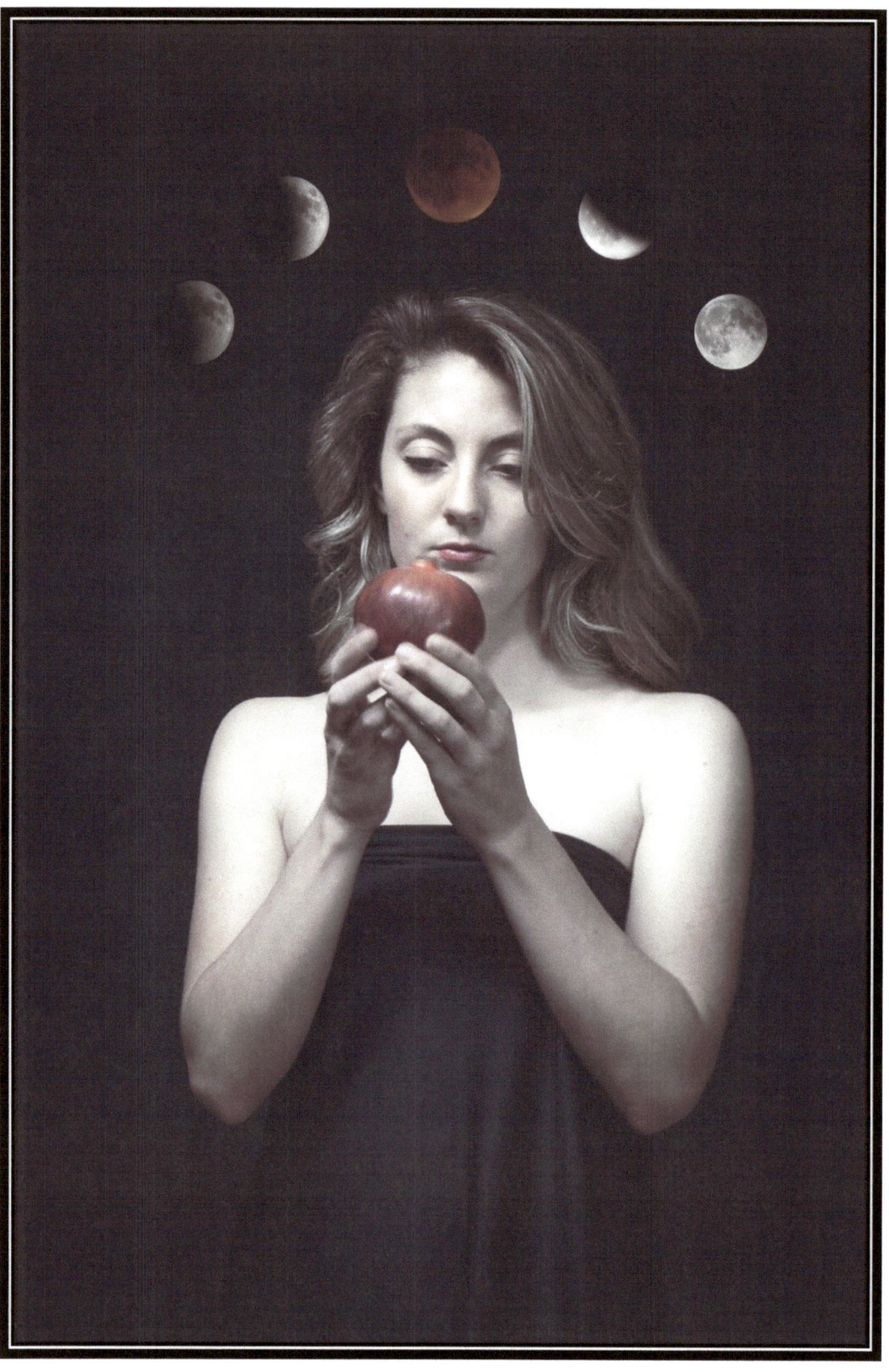

Image 7-3   "Turn, Turn, Turn"

SEEING COLOR COLORBLIND

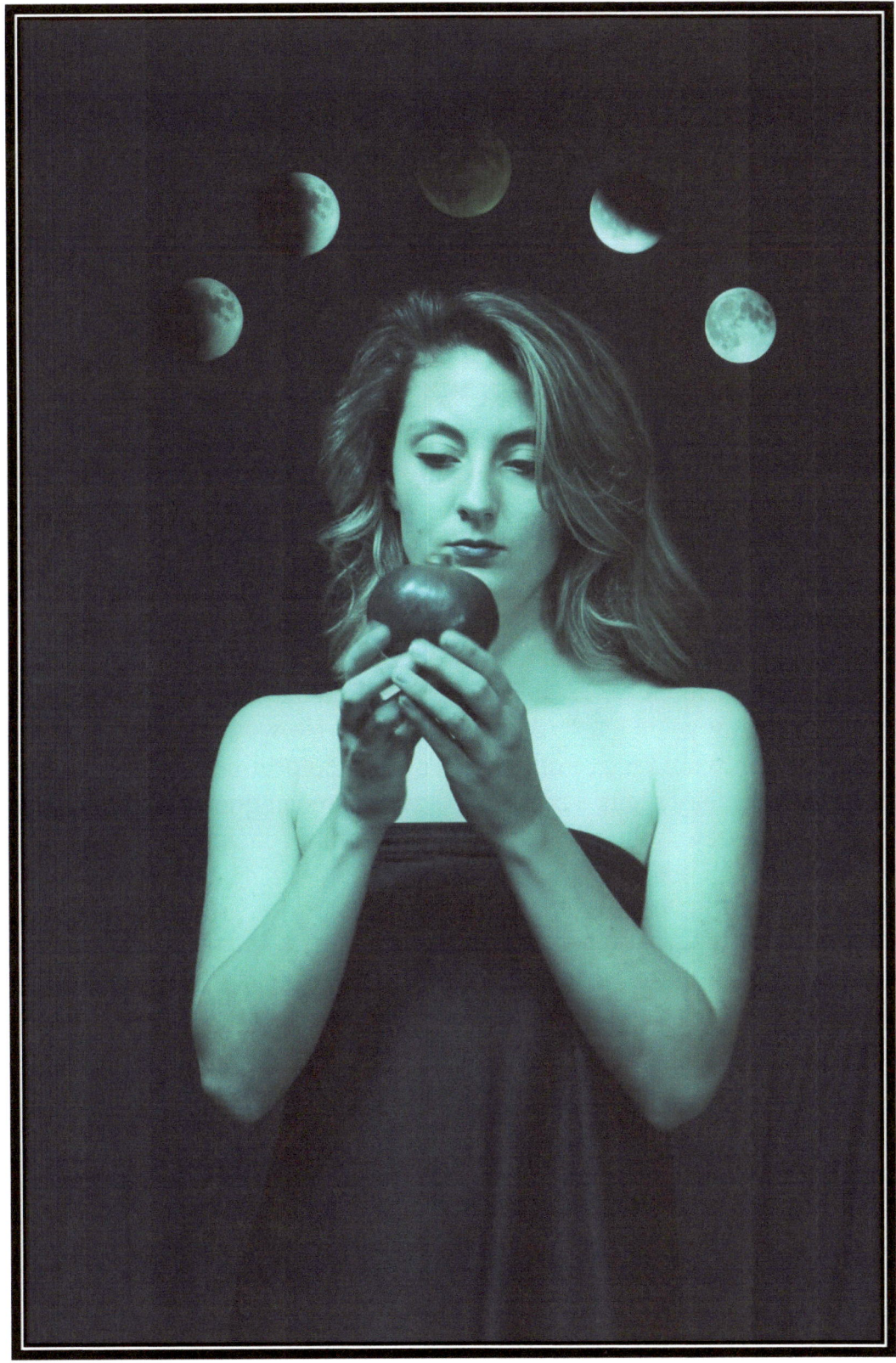

POSTSCRIPT

This project and photo essay on "seeing color colorblind" was very personal to me: my son has and my father had severe red deficiency. Through photography, I was finally able to see the world through their eyes. My son has worked with me to confirm that both images in each of the diptychs appear the same to him. It was a win-win project for all involved.

Family and friends are just trying to understand when they ask someone who sees the world differently, "what do you see? What color is that?" My father, I realize now, many years later, made a joke of it. He would answer something, and the conversation would move on. But to many "colorblind" people, being asked to name what color they see is a catch 22, a trick, a mean question although not meant that way. "Andrew," in one of the Enchroma (enchroma.com) videos said, "Sometimes I wish people could see what I saw."

The images in this volume let me see the world the way my son sees the world. He can show them to people who want to know what he sees. The images are specific to red dichromacy or protanopia. They do not apply to other types or degrees of color deficiencies. But I hope that these images help family and friends of other red dichromats to understand what their friends and loved ones see.

In a larger sense, perhaps it shows that people can honestly see very different "truths."

ABOUT THE AUTHOR

Susan Brandt Graham is an award winning photographic artist who offers a unique view into the creative feminine mind. Formally trained as a social anthropologist (PhD), and board certified Obstetrician and Gynecologist (MD), she has taught Anthropology at the university level and had a private Ob-Gyn practice until retiring. Living in the "Land of Enchantment," she is never at a loss for photographic subjects. Her main interests currently are conceptual photography and photo essays.

Graham creates and uses photographic images to understand and illustrate many varied aspects of life. "Persephone's Choice: Every Woman's Dilemma" combined her background in social anthropology and medicine with conceptual portraiture to discuss "being female" in human society.

In "Seeing Color Colorblind," she uses photography to "see" the world through the eyes of her son and father, both with severe red color deficiencies. Intrigued since the early 1970's with how the two of them could watch a football game on a black and white television and discuss "the blue team and the yellow team," she solved the mystery as she worked on "seeing color colorblind."

You may see more of her work at her website,
http://SusanBGraham.com
And at her Amazon author page
amazon.com/author/grahamsusanbrandt
For permission for use requests, speaker requests, or purchase of individual images, contact
susanbrandtgraham@gmail.

SUSAN BRANDT GRAHAM

www.ingramcontent.com/pod-product-compliance
Lightning Source LLC
Chambersburg PA
CBHW050858180526
45159CB00007B/2719